NUTRITION FOR JUNIOR ATHLETES

A Practical Guide for Parents and Coaches

DR HOWARD HURST

www.proformsportscience.co.uk

Disclaimer: The information presented in this book is for information and education purposes only and does not constitute medical advice. If you have any concerns about the information contained within this book, especially relating to eating disorders and supplement use, consult a medical professional for further advice. Due to the evolution of nutritional sciences, the author reserves the right to change and update information herein based on presentation of new research.

ACKNOWLEDGEMENTS

Thank you to my two little athletes Isobel and Kieran for providing the inspiration for this book. Thanks also to my wife Ruth for her support and putting up with me hiding away late at night and weekends to write this book.

TABLE OF CONTENTS

INTRODUCTION

This book aims to provide a practical nutritional guide to parents and coaches of young children who perform regular physical activity and take part in competitive sport. It will cover what type of foods to eat and drink for optimal performance and provide some example meals to fuel your child. I will also discuss the timing of feeding and hydration around training and competition to enhance performance and recovery, whilst at the same time ensuring adequate nutrition remains available for your young athletes' physiological and cognitive growth and development.

When considering sport and exercise, numerous factors will influence your child's ability to perform effectively. Asked what these factors are, parents and coaches will often state natural ability, training volume, training intensity and time spent practicing specific sport related skills and techniques. A good nutritional plan is rarely at the top of this checklist. Yet, sound nutritional practices can make the difference between a child (and adults for that matter) being a good athlete and a top athlete.

With the wealth of magazines and websites providing advice these days, often misleading and conflicting, if can be difficult for parents and coaches to know what they should and shouldn't be fuelling their young athletes with and when. Likewise, children should not be viewed as miniature adults and therefore nutritional recommendations developed for adults should not be applied to children, as their rate of growth and development and thus nutritional requirements differs to those of adults. The process of child growth and maturation is energy demanding and too often, young athletes fail to consume enough calories on a daily basis to support both growth and competition. Additionally, the foods young children eat are often calorie-rich, but nutrient poor convenience foods including sugary and fatty snacks, as children tend to make food choices based on taste rather than their nutritional value and proposed health benefits. Despite this, some research indicates that while youth diets are not great, youth athletes do at least con-sume more fruit and vegetables than their non-active peers.

So why have I written this book? Well, as a parent to a young swimmer and working full time as a sports nutritionist and sports science lecturer, I've experienced first-hand and understand the challenges parents face in juggling the demands of family life, work commitments and their child's sporting hobbies and the time constraints rushing from one place to another can have on providing nutritious meals and snacks for your child. Parents often have little time other than to grab something quick and easy for their child to eat (often in the car on the way to training or competition). However, with a small amount of pre-planning you can provide a good nutritious diet that will not only support your child's activity, but will also promote growth and long term healthy eating habits. Therefore, it is hoped that this book will provide parents and coaches with the nutritional knowledge to maximise their youth athletes' performance and health.

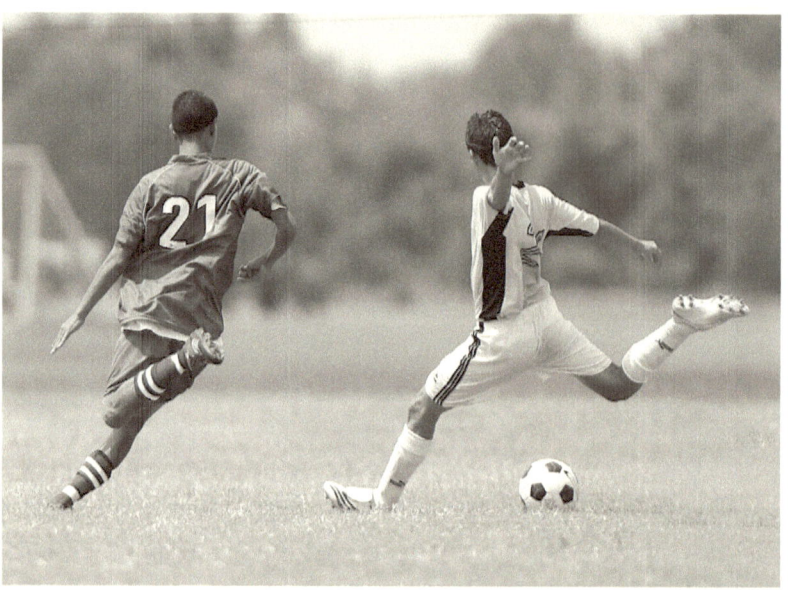

CHAPTER 1: NUTRITION FOR GROWTH

The Developing Athlete

B etween the years of 8 and 18 children's rate of growth increases markedly, particularly around the onset of puberty (typically between 10-14 for girls and 12-16 for boys). There is also wide variability in body shapes and sizes within each age group. Take a look at any group of 12 year olds and you will see huge differences in height, weight, muscular development etc. This process of growth requires lots of energy. Therefore, it is no coincidence that this stage in a child's development also sees a significant increase in appetite. Subsequently, parents and coaches are often concerned about how much they should be feeding their young athletes. However, this will be influenced by numerous factors and will differ child to child, even those of the same age and doing the same sport.

The energy we consume from food and drink and the energy we burn is measured in kilocalories (kcals) and the total daily energy expenditure (TDEE) of a child will be contributed to by three main factors. Firstly, basal metabolic rate (BMR) accounts for roughly 60-75 % of our daily energy expenditure and is the amount of energy the body uses at rest to maintain vital functions such as heart beating, respiration, thermoregulation and brain function. Secondly, the thermic effect of feeding, i.e. the energy required to digest, absorb and transport food and drink, results in around 10 % of TDEE and thirdly, energy expenditure from structured and non-structured physi-cal activity accounts for between 15-30 % of TDEE.[1]

The exact TDEE will also depend on the child's age, body mass, muscularity and the type, intensity and duration of exercise. Additionally, for team sports such as soccer, positional role within the squad will also influ-ence energy requirements, i.e. goalkeepers will require fewer calories dur-ing training and competition than outfield players. Once all of these factors have been accounted for, it is crucial that there is sufficient energy availa-bility remaining to support growth and development. For this reason, TDEE is often much greater than that required by adults. Table 1.1 provides guidelines for the estimated energy requirements of 4 to 18 year olds, though it is important to remember that the more activity the child, the higher the energy requirement will be.[1] While growth rates are very individual, table 1.2 highlights the average gains in body mass and height expected for different age groups and by gender.[2] This can act as a crude guide as to whether your child is developing as expected.

Table 1.1 Estimated energy requirements (kcals) by age, gender and activity level.

	Activity level	Age (years)		
		4-8	9-13	14-18
Male	Sedentary	1400	1800	2200
	Moderately Active	1400-1600	1800-2200	2400-2800
	Very active	1600-2000	2000-2600	2800-3200
Female	Sedentary	1200	1600	1800
	Moderately Active	1400-1600	1600-2000	2000
	Very active	1400-1800	1800-2200	2400

[1]U.S. Department of Agriculture and Department of Health and Human Services. Dietary Guidelines for Americans, 2015.

Table 1.2 Estimated average growth rate and body mass gain by age and gender.

Age (years)	Male		Female	
	Average mass gain (kg/year)	Average height gain (cm/year)	Average mass gain (kg/year)	Average height gain (cm/year)
4-8	1.8 - 2.3	5.1 – 6.4	1.8 - 2.3	5.1 – 6.4
9-13	4.1	6.4*	2.3 - 4.1	6.4*
14-18	19.5	PHV 9.4 - 10.4	9.5	PHV 8.4 – 8.9

PHV = Peak height velocity, the time when a child grows the fastest during their adolescent growth spurt. * differs with onset of puberty.

Energy Cost of Different Sports

As alluded to above, the type of physical activity your child takes part in will influence their caloric needs. Whilst there is much research into energy expenditure for adults across a wide range of sports and activities, the same is not true for children. However, data from Dr Oded Bar-Or, professor of paediatric medicine, provides some estimates for calorie expenditure in children for a limited range of sports.[3] These can be seen in table 1.3 and used in conjunction with the tables above to estimate your young athletes overall energy requirements.

Table1.3 Estimated calorie expenditure (kcals) by body mass (per 10 minutes activity) of children for a range of sports.

Sport	Body Mass (kg)									
	20	25	30	35	40	45	50	55	60	65
Soccer	36	45	54	63	72	81	90	99	108	117
Running										
8 km/h	37	45	52	60	66	72	78	84	90	95
10 km/h	48	55	64	73	79	85	92	100	107	113
Basketball	34	43	51	60	68	77	85	94	102	110
Cycling										
10 km/h	15	17	20	23	26	29	33	36	39	42
15 km/h	22	27	32	36	41	46	50	55	60	65
Tennis	22	28	33	39	44	50	55	61	66	72
Walking										
4 km/h	17	19	21	23	26	28	30	32	34	36
6 km/h	24	26	28	30	32	34	37	40	43	48
Swimming (30m/min)										
Breaststroke	19	24	29	34	38	43	48	53	58	62
Crawl	25	31	37	43	49	56	62	68	74	80
Backstroke	17	21	25	30	34	38	42	47	51	55

3Adapted from: Bar-Or, O. (1983) Pediatric Sports Medicine for the Practitioner.

Sleeping For Success

An often overlooked aspect of growth and development and subsequently the ability to perform and recover well, is sleep. Getting enough 'vitamin Zzzz' is important as it allows the body to recover and adapt to training and competition loads. In addition, research suggests that sleep deprivation may contribute to the increased prevalence of diabetes and/or obesity. This relationship between lack of sleep, weight gain and the risk of diabetes has been suggested to be due in part to 1) altered glucose metabolism[4], 2) increase of appetite[5], and 3) decreased energy expenditure.[6] However, a particular challenge for teenagers is that their biological clock differs to adults and therefore they are often more alert later in the evening. To ensure a good night's sleep, parents should get their children to turn off their mobile phones or computers about an hour before bed, as this has been shown to aid sleep. As a guide, children aged 7 to 12 should aim for 10 to 11 hours sleep per night and children aged 13 to 18 should get between 8 and 9 hours sleep.[7]

References

1. U.S. Department of Agriculture and Department of Health and Human Services. Dietary Guidelines for Americans, 2015. Available at: http://www.health.gov/dietaryguidelines/2015-scientific-report/PDFs/Scientific-Report-of-the-2015-Dietary-Guidelines-Advisory-Committee.pdf.
2. Rogol, AD., Clark, PA. and Roemmich, JN (200) Growth and pubertal development in children and adolescents: effect of diet and physical activity. *The American Journal of Clinical Nutrition*, 72(2), 521S-528S.
3. Bar-Or, O. (1983) Pediatric Sports Medicine for the Practitioner. From: *Physiologic Principles to Clinical Applications*, New York: Springer Verlag.
4. Spiegel, K., Leproult, R. and Van Cauter, E. (1999) Impact of sleep debt on metabolic and endocrine function. *Lancet*, 354,1435–1439.
5. Spiegel, K., Leproult, R., L'Hermite-Baleriaux, M., Copinschi, G., Penev, P. and Van Cauter E. (2004) Leptin levels are dependent on sleep duration: Relationships with sympathovagal balance, carbohydrate regulation, cortisol, and thyrotropin. *Journal of Clinical Endocrinology and Metabolism*, 89, 5762–5771.
6. Weaver, TE., Laizner, AM., Evans, LK., et al. (1997) An instrument to measure functional status outcomes for disorders of excessive sleepiness. *Sleep*, 20, 835–43.
7. How much sleep does my child need? *The Sleep Council*. Available at: https://sleepcouncil.org.uk/how-much-sleep-does-my-child-need/

CHAPTER 2: MACRONUTRIENTS

The energy we derive from food and drink comes primarily from three key nutrients, carbohydrates, proteins and fats. These are commonly referred to as macronutrients and each play different roles within the body. If the balance of these macronutrients is sub-optimal, then exercise performance along with growth will be compromised.

Whilst vitamins and minerals are needed in smaller quantities, they are vital to the metabolism of foods and contribute to hundreds of other functions within the body, such as immune function, wound healing and repairing cellular damage. Collectively these are referred to as micronutrients. However, if a child is provided with a nutritious balanced diet, it is uncommon for vitamin and mineral deficiencies to occur, even in those who are very active.

The general nutrient requirements of athletic youths is not too dissimilar to that of their non-athletic peers or adults. As discussed in chapter 1, it is the quantities of macronutrients that differ. Public Health England updated their Eatwell Guide in 2018, which provides an overview of what the population in general should be consuming with respect to the different macronutrients.[1]

Your young athletes should be aiming for around 45-65 % of their daily nutrients coming from carbohydrates, 25-35 % from healthy fats and 15-30 % from protein. This chapter will provide an overview of the role of these macronutrients and how much your young athletes should be consuming and what the best sources of these nutrients are.

Carbohydrates - Fuelling the Engine

Over the past few years' carbohydrates have come in for a pretty rough time, with seemingly endless condemnation from fitness magazines and online 'experts' who have linked them to diabetes, inflammation, heart dis-ease, obesity and almost everything else in between. This demonisation of carbohydrates has also not been helped by the increase in popularity of diets such as paleo, ketogenic, juicing and low carb-high fat. However, such derision is unjustified.

Carbohydrates are necessary in our diet, as they play a vital role in many of our biological processes. Along with being the primary energy source for moderate to high intensity exercise, they are the exclusive energy source for the nervous system and brain function, help with the production of melatonin and therefore aid sleep and they are actually needed for the metabolism of fats (we'll leave the biochemistry lesson on this for another book). Additionally, they also help maintain concentration during the day, therefore keeping your child more alert at school and during exercise.

The timing of carbohydrate intake needs to take training duration and intensity into account. Increasing intake around training times can help maximise muscle uptake of energy rich foods. It is also not uncommon for young athletes, such as swimmers, to training twice a day for 3 to 4 hours in total. This makes their recovery between sessions vital, as there may be limited time during which muscle glycogen (carbohydrates) stores can be replenished.

However, parents and coaches should be mindful that a child's ability to store carbohydrates is lower than that of adults.[2] This is particularly true of young females.[3] Therefore, whilst a modest increase in carbohydrates prior to and during exercise is recommended, the practice of carbohydrate 'loading' in high quantities, 1 to 2 days prior to harder training sessions or competitions, should be avoided. Instead, carbohydrate containing foods should be consumed at regular intervals throughout the day to maintain stable blood sugar levels.

Parents and coaches should also be aware that youth athletes have a higher reliance on carbohydrate usage *during* exercise than adults. Therefore, regular feeding, with say a 6 % carbohydrate drink, during training and competition lasting longer than 60 minutes is recommended.[4,5] For sessions shorter than 60 minutes, plain water is sufficient if the child has fuelled appropriately prior to the session.

Types of Carbohydrates

The type of carbohydrates found in foods can be categorised as either '*simple*' or '*complex*'. The type will influence how readily available the energy within the foods is for activity. Simple carbohydrates can be further classified as either '*monosaccharides*' or '*disaccharides*'. Monosaccharides are simple one unit sugars e.g. glucose, fructose and galactose. These cannot be broken down into any simpler form. By comparison, disaccharides (e.g. sucrose, maltose and lactose) are made up of a combination of two monosaccharides. For example, regular table sugar is made up of glucose and fructose

Simple carbohydrate are absorbed quickly from the digestive system, resulting in hyperglycemia (elevated blood glucose levels). The body then relies on insulin to move the glucose from the blood to the muscle cells and liver where it is stored as glycogen if it is not used immediately for activity. Simple carbohydrates possess limited nutritional value and tend to be found in processed/refined foods such as cereals, candy, soft drinks, white flour products (e.g. white bread) and table sugar.

However, due to their rapid uptake by the body and thus providing a relatively immediate energy source, some simple carbohydrates at strategic times, such as during exercise and during the recovery from exercise, are beneficial. Despite this, your young athlete should not be consuming these simple carbohydrates all of the time, as any excess that is not used for activity or other metabolic processes can be stored as fat in the cells with prolonged over-consumption, which may lead to increased cholesterol levels and a greater risk of developing obesity.

Conversely, complex carbohydrates can be classified as '*polysaccharides*' and '*oligosaccharides*' and are made up of chains of 3-10 monosaccharides and also contain fibre. Whereas simple carbohydrates are absorbed rapidly, complex carbohydrates take longer to digest and therefore don't raise blood sugar levels as quickly. As a result, foods made up of complex carbohydrates provide a sustained, slower release of energy and have a higher nutritional values.

While most children like sweet foods due to their sugar content, an excessive intake of high sugar foods can replace more nutritious carbohydrates that growing athletes require. Though the occasional sweet treat following a long, hard training session is fine (not after every sessions) this should not be at the expense of a proper post exercise recovery plan. Therefore, most of your child's carbohydrate intake should come from complex sources throughout the day, such as those found in whole-meal breads and cereal, pasta, rice, legumes, spinach vegetables and fibrous fruits such as apples, bananas, oranges and strawberries. However, as stated above, simple carbohydrates can help speed recovery, so if you do give your child a treat, try to go for healthier, possibly homemade, treats rather than overly processed shop bought treats. Additionally, making your own healthy snacks can also be fun to do with your children and help promote a lifelong positive relationship to healthy eating and cooking.

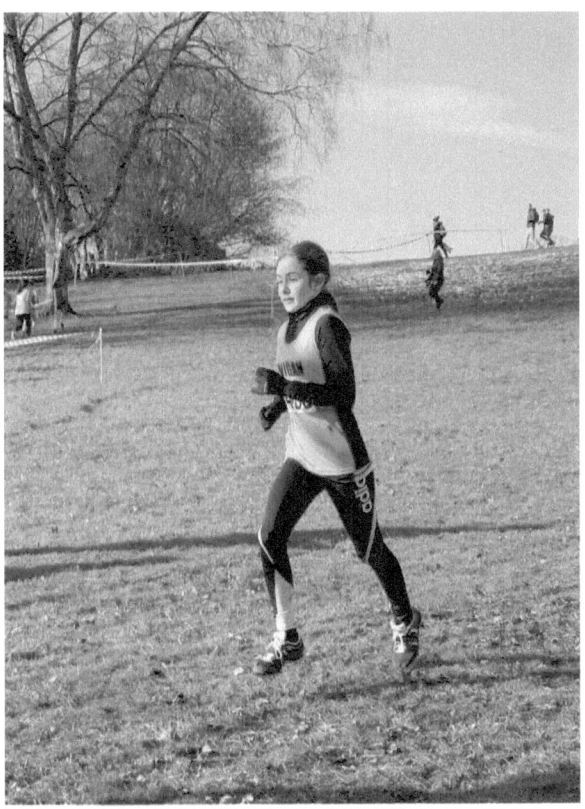

Glycemic Index and Glycemic Load

Exactly how rapidly carbohydrate foods and drinks result in a rise in blood glucose is determined by their glycemic index (GI). This is a scale of 1 to 100 (high GI >70; moderate GI 56-69; low GI <55) and compares how much blood glucose raises following ingestion of a meal or food type compared to when an equal amount of pure glucose is consumed. The higher the GI the quicker the rise in blood glucose, therefore simple carbohydrates tend to have a higher GI, whilst complex carbohydrates have lower GI's due to the slower rise in blood glucose. Table 2.1 provides a list of foods and their respective GI values.

Table 2.1 Average glycemic index of different foods.

Low GI (<55)	Moderate GI (56-69)	High GI (>70)
Apples (36)	Bananas (53)	Glucose (100)
Peanuts (<15)	Maple Syrup (54)	Corn chips (72)
Carrots (35)	Grapes (53)	Watermelon (80)
All bran (42)	Raisins (64)	Honey (73)
Lentils (34)	Orange juice (52)	Bagels (70)
Chickpeas (42)	Porridge oats (58)	Muesli (86)
Pasta (37)	Brown rice (68)	French Fries (75)
Bakes beans (48)	Wholegrain bread (54)	Sports drinks (78)
Peaches 28)	Figs (61)	Bread (white) (79)
Low fat milk (32)	Mango (51)	White rice (72)
Tomatoes (15)	Pineapple (66)	Cornflakes (84)
Kidney beans (26)	Cherries (63)	Pretzels (84)
Sweet potato (44)	Muffin (60)	Baked white potato (85)
Barley (29)	Table sugar (65)	Rice cakes (78)

Whilst GI simply looks at how quickly blood glucose is increased by carbohydrates, glycemic load (GL) also takes into account the actual amount of carbohydrate in a meal/food. To calculate the GL we need to multiply the number of grams (g) of carbohydrate in that food/meal by the GI, then divide this by 100 (maximum attainable GI). For example, from table 2.1 we can see that watermelon has a high glycemic index of 80, therefore it would be logical to assume it will cause blood glucose to rise rapidly. However, in a typical serving size of one-half cup, there is only 5.5 g of carbohydrate. So, the calculated GL is only 4.4 which is low (GL = 5.5*80/100), showing that in actual fact, watermelon is unlikely to cause a significant disturbance in blood sugar or insulin response.

On the other hand a typical 40 g serving of milk chocolate only has a GI of 45 (pretty low) and therefore shouldn't affect blood glucose that much. However, in this serving there are approx. 20 g carbohydrate; therefore 20*45/100 = a GL of 44 (very high) which will result in a rapid increase in blood glucose. Subsequently, insulin levels will increase rapidly to uptake the glucose into the muscles and liver leading to that characteristic hypoglycemic crash many of us have experienced shortly after a candy bar. Figure 2.1 shows the different GI and GL scales.

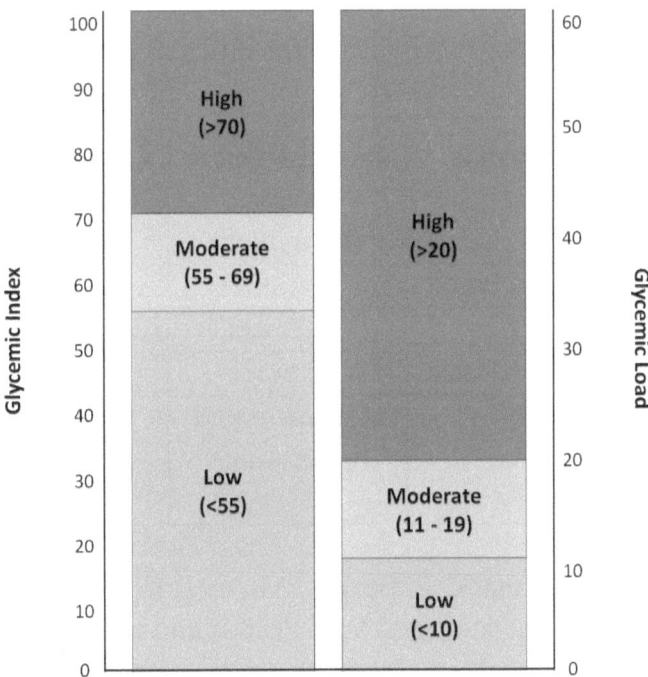

Figure 2.1 Glycemic index versus glycemic load.

Carbohydrate Requirements for Young Athletes

While the general guideline for carbohydrate intake is 45-65 % of total energy intake, the exact amount will vary day to day and will depend on the duration and intensity of exercise and body mass. It is therefore, more accurate to determine the grams of carbohydrate (and protein and fats for that matter) needed per kg of body mass, as it is easily possible to achieve the 45-65 % range, yet be consuming either more or less than the required total calories.

Carbohydrates provide 4 kilocalories (kcals) per gram. Therefore, parents and coaches can easily work out how many grams a child needs based on exercise intensity and multiplying the required grams for a given intensity by their body mass. Table 2.2 outlines the grams of carbohydrate needed for different exercise intensities, whilst table 2.3 provides specific requirements for a range of body masses.

Table 2.2 Carbohydrate requirements for different exercise intensities in young athletes.

Exercise Intensity	Exercise Duration (hours/day)	Carbohydrate requirement (g/kg body mass)
Low intensity/skill based	varied	3-5 g/kg
Moderate intensity	1-2 hours	5-7 g/kg
High intensity/endurance	1-3 hours	6-10 g/kg
Very high intensity	>4 hours or multiple sessions per day	8-12 g/kg

[6] Desbrow B., McCormack, J., Burke, LM., Cox, GR., Fallon, K., Hislop, M. et al., (2014) Sports dieticians Australia position statement: sports nutrition for the adolescent athlete. *International Journal of Sport and Exercise Metabolism*, 24, 570-584.

As an example, if your young athlete is a 12 year old male football player weighing 45 kg, who performs 2 hours of moderate intensity training per day, using table 2.2 we can calculate he needs between 225-315 g of carbohydrate per day. Examples of how, when and what carbohydrates to feed your child will be provided later in this book.

Table 2.3 Carbohydrate requirements (g) for youth athletes by body mass.

Body Mass (kg)	Exercise Intensity			
	Low intensity/skill based	Moderate intensity	High intensity/ endurance	Very high intensity
40	120-200 g	200-280 g	240-400 g	320-480 g
45	135-225 g	225-315 g	270-450 g	360-540 g
50	150-250 g	250-350 g	300-500 g	400-600 g
55	165-275 g	275-385 g	330-550 g	440-660 g
60	180-300 g	300-420 g	360-600 g	480-720 g
65	195-325 g	325-455 g	390-650 g	520-780 g
70	210-350 g	350-490 g	420-700 g	560-840 g

Sources of Carbohydrates

Table 2.4 highlights a range of foods and their typical serving size and the carbohydrate content. Whilst this is not an exhaustive list, it will hopefully help you as a parent or coach to determine how much of various different foods your young athlete needs to consume to achieve their target carbohy-drate intake.

Table 2.4 Carbohydrate content of foods and typical serving size.

	Average serving size (g)	Carbohydrate per average serving (g)
Breads		
Bagel (plain)	85	40
Bread roll (small)	50	25
Bread roll (large)	86	43
Crumpet	46	18
Croissant	48	20
French stick (6")	120	37
Garlic bread (1" slice)	20	10
Sliced bread (medium)	40	17
Sliced bread (thick)	46	19
Naan bread (plain)	73	32
Malt loaf	32	21
Cereals		
Cheerios	30	23
Cornflakes	30	25
Crunchy nut cornflakes	30	24
Frosties	30	26
Muesli (no added sugar)	50	31
Porridge oats	45	30
Shreddies	35	25
Weetabix (2 biscuits)	38	25
Coco Pops	31	27
Main meal items		
Pasta (cooked)	230	73
Rice (cooked)	180	56
Jacket Potato (medium)	180	38
Sweet potato	130	27

Table 2.4 continued.

	Average serving size (g)	Carbohydrate per average serving (g)
Fruit		
Apple	100	11
Banana (medium)	100	23
Fruit cocktail (in juice)	115	17
Grapes (small bunch)	100	15
Mango (1 slice)	40	6
Nectarine (medium)	150	12
Peach (medium)	110	8
Orange (medium)	160	14
Pear	170	16
Pineapple (fresh, 1 ring)	80	12
Vegetables		
Asparagus	180	8
Beetroot	170	17
Broccoli	36	6
Bell pepper	246	15
Carrots	150	15
Cauliflower	100	5
Green beans	125	10
Kale	67	7
Spinach	180	7
Dairy		
Greek yogurt	125	6
Low fat fruit yogurt	125	17
Milk (soya)	200	5
Milk (almond)	200	0.4
Milk (coconut)	200	5.6
Milk (semi-Skimmed)	200	9.6

[7]Diabetes UK (2018) Carbohydrate reference list.

What about Sugar?

Sugar is simply another form of carbohydrate and as such can be used as a useful source of energy for exercise. However, over the last 20 years' manufacturers of sugary snacks and energy drinks have taken this idea and used it in marketing campaigns to claim their products provide more energy for activity and many have even designed packaging specifically to appeal to youngsters. As a result, it is all too common these days to see young athletes chugging down energy drinks and eating sugary foods right before training and competition. Whilst manufacturers aren't necessarily lying, their claims need to be put into context, as the timing of eating such snacks is important in relation to their effectiveness. Consuming high sugar snacks and beverages just before exercise can actually lead to a decrease in perfor-mance, due to the hypoglycemic crash, discussed previously. We will come back to this process in more detail in Chapter 7's '*Why do we need to eat 2 hours before exercise?*'.

While fruit and vegetables also contain sugar, referred to as intrinsic sugars, these tend not to present a major issue with diet and health, as these sugars are bound to the cellular structures of the fruit and vegetables. Instead parents and coaches should monitor consumption of foods with added or free sugar, known as non-milk extrinsic sugar (NMES), such as those found in confectionary, honey, fruit juice and table sugar, as these sugars have being linked to obesity and can also affect dental health due to their high acidity.

Government guidelines recommend that added sugars should contrib-ute no more than 5 % of our daily energy intake. This equates to less than 30 g added sugar (roughly 7 sugar cubes) per day for over 11 year olds and adults, no more than 24 g (~6 sugar cubes) for children aged 7 to 10 and less than 19 g of added sugar (5 sugar cubes) for children aged 4 to 6. Cur-rently, there are no guidelines for sugar intake for under 4 years, though it is recommended sugary foods and drinks be avoided.

One of the problems with trying to determine how much added sugar your child is consuming, is that nutrition labels on packaging rarely state the amount of added sugars. However, the "carbohydrates of which sugars" values on the label can give you a good indication of whether the product is high or low in sugar. This describes the total amount of sugar from all sources, added, from milk and those from the fruit and vegetables. The following thresholds have been set to classify food and drink sugar levels:

- More than 22.5 g of sugar per 100 g is considered high and often coloured red on the label
- Between 5 and 22.5 g of sugar per 100 g is deemed moderate, coloured amber on label
- Less than 5 g of sugar per 100 g is considered low, coloured green on label

Bear in mind not all labels will colour code their labels. Sometimes labels only present a single figure for carbohydrates and not a value for the 'of which sugar'. This makes it more difficult to determine how much free/added sugar is in the products. In these cases you will need to look at the ingredients list and look for words such as high-fructose corn syrup, corn syrup, sucrose, glucose, crystalline sucrose, nectar, agave, molasses etc. These are all other names for types of sugar and should be limited in your child's diet.

Protein - Building Blocks for Growth and Development

Protein is one of the most debated macronutrients over the past decade, with magazines and websites touting it as a wonder nutrient. However, while there is no question that protein is important, like most other things within the body, it is tightly regulated. Therefore, consuming additional protein above an individual's requirements isn't necessarily healthy, especially for children. Once the protein requirements have been met, any excess will either be used as fuel or be broken down and excreted in the urine, which may place additional stress on the kidneys and liver. Research has also shown that children in most developed Western countries already consume sufficient protein from a balanced diet, whilst athletic children get two to three times their protein needs daily.[8]

Still, taking protein supplements or adding protein powders to foods, shakes or smoothies is an increasing trend seen in children. This is especially true of young athletic children and particularly boys who wants to bulk up and get bigger and stronger. However, simply consuming more protein than is necessary will not build more muscle. Muscular development will only occur as a result of consistent training.

While it may be convenient and quicker to provide your young athlete with a protein supplement post-training, with a small amount of forward planning parents and coaches should be able to ensure their children are getting their protein requirements from real foods without having to rely on supplements. However, there are times when a supplement may be appropriate, such as if real foods are not readily available soon after competition if travelling away or where a child may be struggling to meet their protein needs through diet alone.

While protein is not used as a primary source of energy, like carbohydrates, it too provides 4 kcals of energy per gram. However, it is used more so for the building and repairing of muscle tissue, producing thousands of hormones, some of which are required for the metabolism of carbohydrates and fats, strengthening skin and bones, transporting nutrients and is also involved in supporting immune functions.

Protein is made up of 20 smaller compounds called amino acids. Of these, 11 are known as *non-essential amino acids*, which are produced naturally within the body and 9 are classified as *essential amino acids*, as they are not produced by the body and therefore must come from our diet. Of the essential amino acids, leucine, isoleucine and valine, referred to as *branched chain amino acids*, are of particular importance, as they have been shown to be involved in muscle protein synthesis.[9]

The two main types of dairy protein are *whey* and *casein*. Whey is faster acting and results in a greater amino acid spike and therefore a greater degree of muscle protein synthesis due to its high leucine content. However, it is relatively short lasting, hence it is better immediately following exercise. Casein protein on the other hand, is slower acting and stays in the body much longer, therefore it provides a better source of protein prior to bed to work overnight to supply amino acids. For vegetarian and vegan athletes, good alternative sources of protein are lentils, nuts, pulses and cereals. However, protein content is lower than in animal products.

Protein Requirements for Young Athletes

Young athletes should aim for between 15-30 % of total daily calorie intake from protein, though for the majority of time, intakes at the lower end of this range will be sufficient. However, this again will be influenced by body mass and also exercise intensity; for example, protein requirement during the start of the season or at the beginning of a training programme may be higher due to the greater demands during that period of training and the greater initial increases in muscle mass seen in the early phases of a training programme. Later in the season when the athlete enters a '*maintenance*' phase, protein intake can be reduced slightly.

As protein is important for growth and development, the protein requirements of athletic youths is greater than that of their non-athletic peers and adults. Whilst protein intake needs to meet the requirements for the rapid growth period that occurs around puberty in both athletic and non-athletic children, young athletes grow at a greater rate and increase muscle mass to a greater extent; therefore, their protein intake needs to account for this and to a smaller degree provide some fuel for exercise.

Typically, the average adult requires around 0.8-1.0 g/kg body mass protein per day, while non-athletic children have been shown to require around 1.2 g/kg.[10] However, whilst data for athletic children is limited, several studies have shown that the protein requirements of young athletes is greater still and should be around 1.4-1.7 g/kg body mass.[11,12] Additionally, one study reported that young athletes engaging in weight lifting or heavy resistance training may require protein intakes as high as 3.4 g/kg, though for the vast majority of young athletes this is unnecessary.[2] Table 2.5 provides some guidelines on how much protein is required for different body masses based on the 1.4-1.7 g/kg recommendations.

Table 2.5 Protein recommendations for young athletes of different body mass.

Body mass (kg)	Protein range (g)
45	63 - 77
50	70 - 85
55	77 - 94
60	84 - 102
65	91 - 111
70	98 - 119

Timing of Protein Intake

The timing of protein ingestion is also important to its function. Young athletes should aim to consume protein with breakfast, as this has been shown to promote whole-body net protein balance, which is a prerequisite for growth.[13] Following this, protein should be eaten every 3 to 4 hours throughout the day.

Additionally, protein intake before and within 2-3 hours immediately post exercise has been shown to speed recovery.[13,14] Therefore, athletes should try to consume around 15-20 grams (0.33 to 0.44 g/kg body mass) as soon after training or competition as possible. This can easily be gained from a large glass of whole milk, which is a good source of whey protein, and a large banana. Prior to going to bed consuming either 200 ml of whole milk*, 100 g of cottage cheese or 150 g of Greek yogurt will provide a good source of casein protein (around 11-15 g). As mentioned previously, there is no need for specific sports recovery drinks with children in this age group.

*Note: milk is a good source of both whey and casein protein, so can work both immediately after exercise and later at night. However, it's worth noting that casein makes up around 82% of the proteins in milk, while whey makes up the remaining 18%.

Sources of Protein

Children generally get enough daily protein if they consume two servings of dairy, such as milk, yogurt, cheese, and one or two servings of lean protein, such as lean beef, pork, poultry and fish. Table 2.6 shows the protein content of various foods by average portion size.

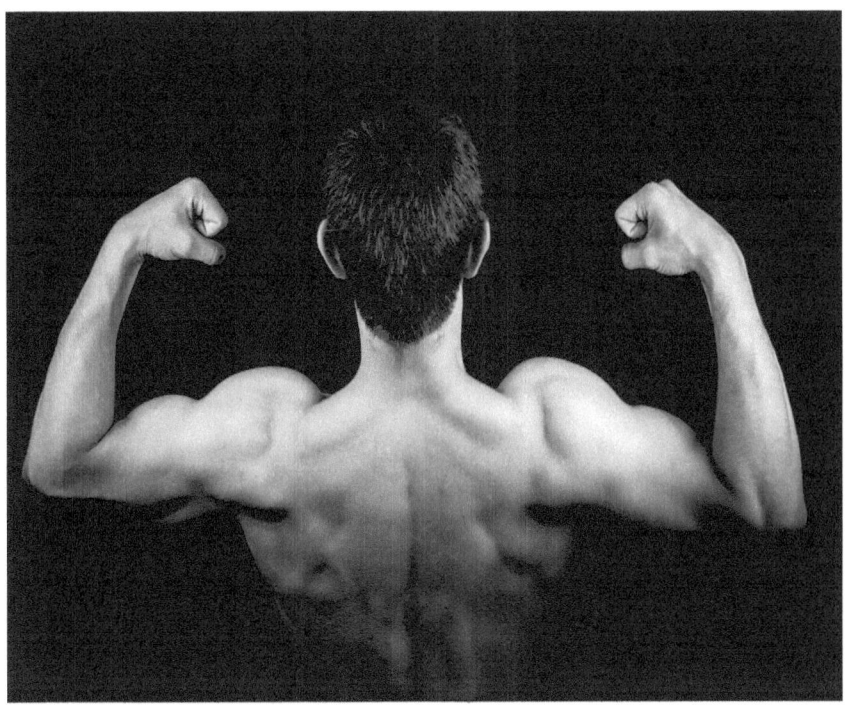

Table 2.6 Protein content of foods and typical serving size.

	Average serving size (g)	Protein per average serving (g)
Meat & Seafood		
Chicken (no skin)	110	32
Steak	100	31
Pork	100	32
Ham	85	14
Lamb chop	100	29
Salmon (filet)	150	30
Tuna (canned)	100	24
Dairy and Eggs		
Eggs (large)	1	6
Greek yogurt	150	15
Yogurt (regular or low fat)	150	6
Cottage cheese	110	11
Milk (whole)	200	7
Milk (Semi-skimmed)	200	7
Milk (Semi-skimmed)	200	7
Milk (Skimmed)	200	3.4
Milk (Soy)	200	7
Cheddar chees	30	8
Legumes and Nuts		
Lentils	113	9
Kidney & Black beans	113	8
Hummus	85	7
Peanut butter 2 (tbsp)	28	7
Sunflower seeds	28	5
Edamame	78	8

Table 2.6 continued.

Grains & Vegetables		
Bread (1 slice)	35	3
Cereal	113	3
Rice	150	4
Pasta	200	10
Peas (green)	113	4
Spinach	113	3
Others		
Tofu	124	10
Quorn mince	75	11

Fats - They're Not All Bad

Fat has gained a bad reputation over the last few decades, but we all need some fat in our diet and athletic youths are no exception. Along with being the main energy source for low to moderate intensity exercise (it provides 9 kcals of energy per gram, compared to 4 kcals per gram carbohydrate and protein), it is also essential for a number of other roles within the body, including creating nerve tissue (including the brain), production of hormones, aiding the absorption of fat soluble vitamins (A, D, E and K), supplying essential fatty acids (omega-3 and omega-6) which are not produced by the body naturally, therefore must come from food intake, promotes immune function, help regulate body temperature, helps prevent fatigue[15] and provides cushioning around the organs to protect against injury.

Children have also been shown to rely more on fat stores than carbohydrates relative to adults (remember, children don't store carbohydrates so well).[15] Therefore, 'good' fats are required to fuel lower intensity exercise lasting greater than 60 minutes.

Types of Fats

Fats are generally classified as either '*unsaturated*' or '*saturated*' depending on their chemical composition. Saturated fats are often seen as the 'bad' fats, as they have been shown to lead to increases in low-density lipoproteins (LDL) cholesterol (the bad ones), whilst unsaturated fats are seen as the 'good' fats, as they promote increases in high-density lipoproteins (HDL) cholesterol (the good ones). However, it is not that simple, as research over the last few years has found that not all saturated fats are bad for us. For example, lauric acid is a saturated fat found in high quantities in coconut oil and is known to increase HDL cholesterol, therefore having a positive effect on the total:HDL cholesterol ratio and therefore health*.[16] As a result, it probably more appropriate to look at healthy food types rather than fat types when deciding what your young athlete should be eating.

NOTE: *it should be noted that where coconut oil is concerned, there is still debate as to the health benefits of the lauric acid in it, as some studies have shown that while HDL cholesterol is increased, it may not function as expected, therefore having minimal positive benefits to health.*

Fat Requirements for Young Athletes

The recommended daily intake of total fats for adults and children should be between 25-35 % of their total daily calories, or up to 95 g depending on body mass and total calorie intake. For saturated fat, intake should be less than 30 g for adult males, less than 20 g for females and for child it should be between 20-27 g. Whilst there are no specific guidelines for young athletes and whilst we now know not all saturated fats are bad, it is still recommended that these children get the bulk of their fat intake from unsaturated fats, while their intake of saturated fats (mainly from animal fats) and trans fats (found in highly processed foods, such as margarines, cookies, fast food etc.) should be limited as much as possible, preferably to less than 10 % of total daily calories.

Sources of Fats

When planning your athletes' diet, try to include healthy fats from sources such as oily fish like salmon and mackerel, eggs, nuts, seeds and avocados. Reduced fat dairy products such as low fat milk, cheese and yoghurt can be given to children over 4, though check the food labels for excess sugar and salt, as these are often added to low fat option to maintain taste. However, for active children, this isn't particularly necessary and full fat dairy products are fine. Table 2.7 presents examples of both healthy and unhealthy foods and the fat content in a typical serving.

Table 2.7 Fat content of foods and typical serving size.

	Average serving size (g)	Fat per average serving (g)
Healthy fats (eat often)		
Almonds	28	14
Avocados (1 whole)	200	29
Coconut Oil (1 tbsp)	15	14
Eggs (1 whole)	50	5
Extra virgin olive oil	15	14
Mackerel (1 filet)	176	18
Almond butter (1 tbsp)	15	9
Nuts	30	16
Olives (6 green olives)	15	5
Salmon (1 filet cooked)	143	12
Unhealthy fats (eat occasionally)		
Ice Cream (vanilla)	66	7
Crisps	35	12
French fries (medium serving)	117	17
Hamburger	95	8
Margarine (1 tbsp)	15	11
Milk chocolate (1 bar)	44	13
Muffin (1 medium)	113	18
Pizza (1 slice)	107	10

References

1. Eatwell Guide (2018) *Public Health England.* Available at: https://assets.publishing.service.gov.uk/government/uploads/syste m/uploads/attachment_data/file/742750/Eatwell_Guide_booklet_2 018v4.pdf

2. Hoch, AZ., Goossen, K. and Kretschmer, T. (2008) Nutritional requirements of the child and teenage athlete. *Physical Medicine and Rehabilitation clinics of North America*, 19, 373-398.

3. Position of the American Dietetic Association, Dieticians of Canada, and the American College of Sports Medicine (2009): Nutrition and Athletic Performance. *Journal of the* Academy *of* Nutrition *and Dietetics*, 109, 509-527.

4. Riddell, MC., Bar-Or, O., Schwarcz, HP. and Heigenhauser, GJF. (2000) Substrate utilisation in boys during exercise with [13C]-glucose ingestion. *European Journal of Applied Physiology*, 83, 441-448.

5. Phillips, SM., Turner, AP., Gray, S., Sanderson, MF. and Spoule, J. (2010) Ingesting 6% carbohydrate-electrolyte solution improves endurance capacity, but not sprint performance, during intermittent, high-intensity shuttle running in adolescent team games players aged 12-14 years. *European Journal of Applied Physiology*, 109(5), 811-821.

6. Desbrow B., McCormack, J., Burke, LM., Cox, GR., Fallon, K., Hislop, M. et a., (2014) Sports dieticians Australia position statement: sports nutrition for the adolescent athlete. *International Journal of Sport and Exercise Metabolism*, 24, 570-584.

7. Diabetes UK (2018) Carbohydrate reference list. Available at: https://www.diabetes.org.uk/resources-s3/2017-11/carb-reference-list-0511.pdf

8. Jeukendrup, A. and Cronin, L. (2011) Nutrition and elite young athletes. *Medicine and Science in Sport and Exercise*, 56, 47-58.

9. Tang, JE., Moore, DR., Kujbida, GW., Tarnopolsky, MA. and Phillips, SM. (2009) Regulation of protein metabolism in exercise and recovery ingestion of whey hydrolysate, casein, or sot protein

isolate: effects on mixed muscle protein synthesis at rest and following resistance exercise in young men. *Journal of Applied Physiology*, 107, 987-992.

10. Bar-Or, O. (2000) Nutrition for child and adolescent athletes. *Sports Science Exchange*, 77.

11. Aerenhouts, D., Van Cauwenberg, J., Poortmans, JR., Hauspie, R. and Clarys, P. (2013) Influence of growth rate on nitrogen balance in adolescent sprint athletes. *International Journal of Sport Nutrition and Exercise Metabolism*, 23(4), 409-417.

12. Boisseau, N., Creff, C., Loyens, M. and Poortmans, JR. (2002) Protein intake and nitrogen balance in male non-active adolescents and soccer players. *European Journal of Applied Physiology*, 88(3), 288-293.

13. Karagounis, LG., Volterman, KA., Breuille, D., Offord, EA., Emady-azar, S. and Moore, DR. (2018) Protein intake at breakfast promotes a positive whole-body protein balance in a dose response manner in healthy children: A randomised trial. *Journal of Nutrition*, 148, 729-737.

14. Phillips, SM., Moore, DR. and Tang, JE. (2007) A Critical Examination of Dietary Protein Requirements, Benefits, and Excesses in Athletes. *International Journal of Sport Nutrition and Exercise Metabolism*, 17(1), 58-76.

15. Butte, NF. (2000) Fat intake of children in relation to energy requirements. *The American Journal of Clinical Nutrition*, 72, 1246s-1252s.

16. Dayrit, FM. (2015) The properties of lauric acid and their significance in coconut oil. *Journal of American Oil Chemists' Society*, 92, 1-15.

CHAPTER 3: MICRONUTRIENTS

There are a broad range of vitamins and minerals, all of which play different, but vital roles in maintaining health and aid growth and development. These nutrients are collectively known as '*micronutrients*', as they are required in much smaller quantities than carbohydrates, fats and proteins. Whilst most people accept micronutrients are a requirement for health, their specific function and need are often overlooked. Unlike macronutrients, they do not provide energy directly, but are required in the production of energy from macronutrients. In addition, they are also involved in muscle function, brain function, development of muscle and nerve tissue, red blood cell production and maintaining healthy bones to name a few.

Types of Vitamins

Vitamins can be categorised as either '*fat-soluble*' or '*water-soluble*'. Fat-soluble vitamins (A, D, E and K) are absorbed by the small intestine and as they do not dissolve in water, they are stored in fatty tissue and the liver. However, in high doses these vitamins can become toxic, and whilst toxicity is rare, they can cause liver and bone damage, irregular heart beat and elevated blood pressure if consumed in excessive amounts.

Water-soluble vitamins, such as the B vitamins, vitamin C, thiamin, biotin and choline, are dissolved in water both within the body and during cooking processes, therefore their storage within the body is very low. As a result, your young athlete needs to consume these through diet on a daily basis. Also, unlike fat-soluble vitamins, if an athlete consumes too much of a water-soluble vitamin, the excess is simply excreted from the body via the urine. Subsequently, toxicity from these vitamins is extremely rare.

Influence of Cooking Method on Vitamin and Mineral Content

The way we cook our food will also influence its nutrient content. Though cooking our food can help to improve its digestion and increases absorption of many nutrients, the way in which we cook food can dramatically reduce vitamin and mineral levels. For example, as water-soluble vitamins dissolve when in water, boiling, poaching and simmering foods will reduce the amounts of these vitamins available for function within the body. Therefore, dry cooking methods, such as grilling, stir-frying and microwaving can help retain more of the vitamins and minerals in our food.

Vitamin and Mineral Requirements for Young Athletes

In the UK the Scientific Advisory Committee on Nutrition (SACN) (www.sacn.org.uk) have determined the reference nutrient intake (RNI) for many of these vitamins and minerals. The RNI is the average amount of a nutrient considered sufficient to meet the needs of 97 % of the population. However, while these RNI's don't necessarily account for the greater needs of athletes and in particular young athletes, ensuring you child consumes a balanced diet with enough fruit and vegetables is sufficient to make sure they are getting enough vitamins and minerals to support their needs, without relying on supplements. Table 3.1 and table 3.2 details the RNI's of vitamins and minerals for children in the UK.

Table 3.1 UK Reference Nutrient Intakes for vitamins for children.

Gender	Age (Years)				
	7-10	11-14		15-48	
	Male & Female	Males	Females	Males	Females
Vitamin A (µg/day)	500	600	600	700	600
Thiamin (mg/day)	0.7	0.9	0.7	1.1	0.8
Riboflavin (mg/day)	1.0	1.2	1.1	1.3	1.1
Niacin equivalent (mg/day)	12.0	15	12	15	14
Vitamin B_6 (mg/day)	1.0	1.2	1.0	1.2	1.2
Vitamin B_{12} (µg/day)	1.0	1.2	1.2	1.2	1.5
Folate (µg/day)	150	200	200	200	200
Vitamin C (mg/day)	30	35	35	40	40
Vitamin D (µg/day)	10	10	10	10	10

Note: Vitamin requirements for 7-10 year olds are the same for both genders.

Table 3.2 UK Reference Nutrient Intakes for minerals for children.

Gender	7-10 Male & Female	11-14 Males	11-14 Females	15-48 Males	15-48 Females
Calcium (mg/day)	550	1000	800	1000	800
Chloride (mg/day)	1800	2500	2500	2500	2500
Copper (mg/day)	0.7	0.8	0.8	1.0	1.0
Iodine (µg/day)	110	130	130	140	140
Iron (mg/day)	8.7	11.3	14.8	11.3	14.8
Magne-sium (mg/day)	200	280	280	300	300
Phospho-rous (mg/day)	450	775	625	775	625
Potassium (mg/day)	2000	3100	3100	3500	3500
Sodium (mg/day)	1200	1600	1600	1600	1600
Selenium (µg/day)	30	45	45	70	60
Zinc (mg/day)	7	9	9	9.5	7

Note: Mineral requirements for 7-10 year olds are the same for both genders.

Vitamins and Their Functions

Vitamin A is needed for growth and development and is important for healthy vision, particularly in low light. It is also required to keep skin, hair and the linings of many organs healthy, and as an antioxidant it is involved in the immune system to help fight illness and infections. However, excess vitamin A, as a result of too many supplements, can lead to liver and bone damage in children due it being stored in the body's fat. The best sources of vitamin A are liver, eggs, cheese, butter/margarine, oily fish, fruit and vegetables. However, as many animal feeds are now enriched with vitamin A and subsequently liver has high levels, it is recommended liver is only eaten once per week.

B vitamins include riboflavin, thiamin, niacin, biotin, folate, pyridoxine, pantothenic acid and vitamin B_{12}. They are all needed for the development of the nervous system and for the conversion of food to energy. In addition, vitamin B_{12} and folate can help to prevent the development of anaemia. The best sources of folate are dark green vegetables, liver and pulses, whilst good sources of the other B vitamins are meat, dairy products, eggs, cereals, seeds and fish.

Vitamin C is need is required to form collagen and connective tissues within the body and helps maintain healthy bones, teeth and gums, blood vessels and immune function. It is also needed to aid the absorption of iron. Fruits such as blackcurrants, raspberries, oranges and kiwi and vegetables such as broccoli, cabbage, tomatoes and peppers are all excellent sources of vitamin C.

Vitamin D is necessary for the absorption of calcium and maintenance of calcium levels in the blood and bones and may help prevent osteoporosis in later life. However, getting enough vitamin D can be challenging for those living in the Northern Hemisphere. Vitamin D is sometimes referred to as the 'sunshine vitamin', as exposure to sunlight helps to synthesis vitamin D within the skin. However, due to a reduction in daylight hours over the winter months and spending less time outdoors, the synthesis of vitamin D can be limited. Despite this, spending time outside everyday over the summer months can help build up sufficient stores of vitamin D to last the winter months. There are several other factors that can influence vitamin D production, including excessive coverage of skin with clothing (as the sun needs direct exposure to the skin for production of vitamin D), skin colour (those with darker skin pigment do not produce as much vitamin D) and environmental conditions such as cloud cover and pollution will also reduce the strength of the sunlight and therefore limit vitamin D production. Exposure to sunlight is the best source of vitamin D, as few foods have significant levels, though oily fish, eggs, liver and fortified cereals do provide small amounts.

Vitamin E is an antioxidant that has been shown to protect against heart disease. It is also needed to promote normal cell growth and development. Sources of vitamin E include vegetable oils, butter, avocados, meat, oily fish and eggs.

Vitamin K is needed to ensure our blood clots normally following a cut or injury. Vitamin K1 (phylloquinone) is found mainly in leafy green vegetables and soybean, whilst vitamin K2 (menaquinone) is produced by bacteria in the intestines.

Minerals and Their Functions

Calcium is need for the development of strong bones and teeth and many people are aware of these roles. However, calcium is also important to ensure proper blood clotting and is needed for the contraction of heart muscle and skeletal muscles. Dairy products such as milk, yogurt and cheese are the best sources of calcium, though other sources also include dark green leafy vegetables, legumes, nuts and seeds and sardines. For vegetarians soya milk can be consumed, though this must be fortified with extra calcium.

Iodine is a key component in the hormone thyroxine, which helps to convert food to energy and promote physical and mental development. Iodine deficiency can be a problem in some parts of Europe, though this is less common in the UK, as farming methods mean British milk is a good source of iodine. Other sources of iodine include eggs, fish, wholegrains, green beans, courgettes, kale, spring greens, watercress, strawberries and potatoes with the skin on.

Iron is important for the formation of red blood cells and haemoglobin and therefore the transportation of oxygen in the blood. As mentioned previously, it is also important for the prevention of anaemia. Young female athletes particularly should have their iron levels checked regularly, as iron losses are increased during menstruation and these losses are comparable to those reported in adult females.[2] However, the amount of iron lost during menstruation is highly variable, but iron intake should still be increase around this time. One study suggested an increase in daily iron intake of approximately 2.1 mg/day are required to offset menstrual losses.[2] Iron in our food comes in two forms: the readily absorbed '*haem iron*' found in red meats, pork, lamb, poultry and fish, and the less well absorbed (requiring the presence of vitamin C for absorption) '*non-haem iron*'. This is found in fortified breakfast cereals, eggs, pulses, fruit and some vegetables.

Sodium is required in the diet for helping to maintain fluid balance and blood pressure and is the main electrolyte added to sports drinks. It contributes to hydration by stimulating thirst, promoting increased fluid intake, enhancing fluid absorption and replacing sodium lost in sweat. The primary source of sodium is salt, which is found in many foods as a preservative. Sodium levels are also high in many processed foods and snacks to enhance flavour, therefore these should be limited for your young athletes.

Zinc is beneficial for a healthy immune system and helps with the growth of skin cells. It is also required for wound healing. The best sources of zinc are eggs, meat, wholegrain cereals and dairy products.

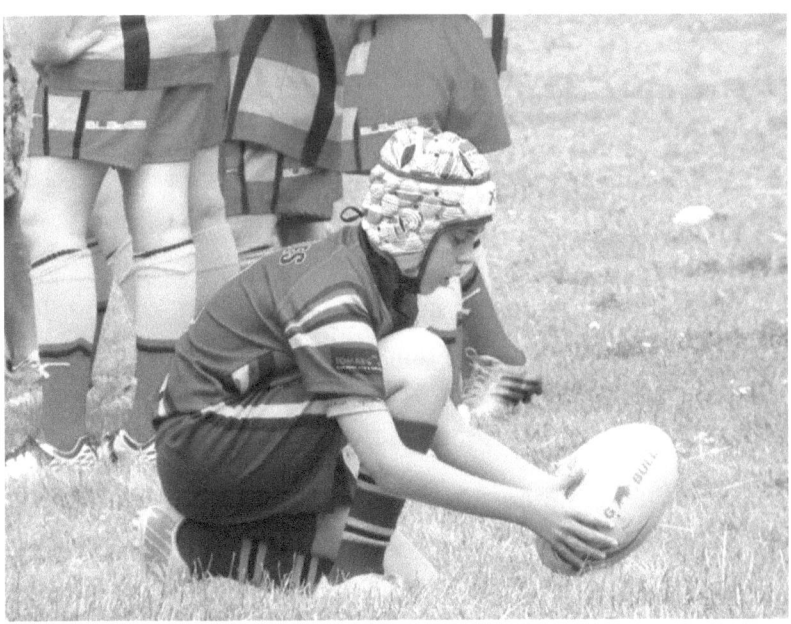

References

1. Government dietary recommendations: Government recommendations for energy and nutrients for males and females aged 1-18 years and 19+ years. (2016) Available at: https://assets.publishing.service.gov.uk/government/uploads/syste m/uploads/attachment_data/file/618167/government_dietary_reco mmendations.pdf

2. Hallberg, L. (1996) Iron requirements, iron balance and iron deficiency in menstruating and pregnant women. Hallberg, L. Asp, N-G. eds. *Iron Nutrition in Health and Disease*, 165-182, John Libbey and Co.

CHAPTER 4: HYDRATION FOR PERFORMANCE

Why Is Hydration Important?

P roper hydration is just as important as food intake, both for health and performance. It helps maintain blood pressure, blood volume, the correct balance of electrolytes, prevents dehydration and also aids the transport of nutrients to the muscles cells.

Individual fluid requirements vary widely and are largely dependent on the type and volume of exercise (including both structured activities like training, but also general play during the day at school), and environmental conditions. Unlike most adults, children are often not as aware of how much fluids they have lost through activity and how much they need. For example, young swimmers often fail to notice how much they sweat while swimming due to not being able to see or feel that sweat as a result of being in the pool.

As children are often not conscious enough of fluid needs to maintain good hydration strategies, parents and coaches need to encourage them to drink regularly in order to stay hydrated during training and competition *and* on a daily basis. While it may seem somewhat obvious that this is important during warmer summer months, it is also equally important during winter. Whilst sweat rates may be reduced in colder weather, breathing in cold air can dry out the throat, leading the body to rely on fluid drawn from within the body to moisten that air, which can lead to dehydration. As a result, fluid intake should be increased during colder weather.

Fluid losses will also vary daily depending on several factors such as age, gender, body size exercise type etc. Therefore, your child's fluid intake should be monitored and adjusted accordingly depending upon these and environmental condition, training load and health status.

Hydration and Thermoregulation

Thermoregulation is the body's way of controlling internal temperature and getting rid of excess heat. This is achieved via a number of mechanisms including *evaporation* (heat loss through the conversion of water to gas; evaporation of sweat), *radiation* (heat loss from one object to another, without direct physical contact), *conduction* (heat loss through physical contact with another object or body) and *convection* (heat loss via movement of air or water across the skin). Sweating is an important means of losing heat during exercise, therefore adequate fluid intake to offset these losses is crucial.

Children have long been thought to be at greater risk of heat stress than adults, particularly in hot and/or humid climates, due to physiological and anatomical differences, including a lower sweat capacity, lower economy during exercise, and a greater percentage of blood flow from the heart (cardiac output) being directed to the skin to aid cooling for a given exercise work load. In addition, children have a higher body surface area to body mass ratio, a major factor in "dry" heat dissipation and effective sweat evaporation. However, recent studies directly comparing adults and children have found that with the exception of during extreme heat, children are in fact equally as efficient at controlling body temperature as adults during exercise, despite reduced sweating rates.[1,2]

Sweat rate is also dependent upon age, gender and the stage of puberty. Young males aged 9 years were shown to have sweat rates approximately half that of men aged 21-27 years (455 ml and 815 ml per hour, respectively).[3] In contrast, young females do not appear to have sweat rates different to their young male counterparts or adult females.[4]

Monitoring Hydration Status

It is important to check your young athletes hydration status regularly during training, as decreases in body mass due to fluid loss can lead to impaired athletic performance. Luckily, there are a number of methods for assessing your child's hydration level relatively easily, including use of colour urine charts, monitoring body mass and urine specific gravity.

Urine Colour Charts

A quick guide to hydration is the colour of your child's urine. Urine colour charts use an 8 point colour scale and indicate the quantity of a compound called '*urochrome*', a by-product of the breakdown of haemoglobin. If large amounts of urine are passed, urochrome is also excreted in large amounts, giving urine a pale colour. Conversely, when smaller amounts of urine are passed, urochrome is more concentrated, giving urine a darker colour.[5]

If you notice your child's urine is a darker colour than usual, it is a fair indicator of dehydration and extra fluids should be taken on. Ideally, urine should be a very pale yellow colour. However, care should be taken interpreting these colour charts, as some compound such as B vitamins, carotene, betacyanins found in beetroot can make urine appear darker. Figure 4.1 shows an example of a urine colour chart.

URINE COLOUR CHART
How hydrated am I?

1	**HYDRATED**
2	If your urine is within the colours of 1, 2 & 3 you are well hydrated and should continue to drink as you are.
3	
4	**DEHYDRATED**
5	If your urine colour is between 4 and 6 you are dehydrated and should drink between 1-2 glasses and 1/2 litre of water now.
6	
7	**SEVERELY DEHYDRATED**
8	If your urine is the colour of 6 or 7 you need to drink 1 litre of water immediately.

Figure 4.1 Urine colour chart.

Monitoring Body Mass

Monitoring changes in body mass can also provide a reasonable indicator of hydration status and can be used to determine sweat rates and therefore fluid needs. Sweat loss can be calculated using the following equation:

$$Sweat\ loss\ =\ (body\ mass\ before - body\ mass\ after) + fluid\ intake - urine\ volume$$

Where:

body mass = mass measured before and after exercise;

fluid intake = fluids consumed during training in ml;

and urine volume = ml of urine passed after exercise.

To determine sweat rate, you then simply divide sweat loss by however many minutes or hours of exercise were completed. However, as a slightly rougher general guideline, 1 kg of body mass lost is equal to roughly 1 litre of fluid lost. Your young athlete should then aim to replace 1.5 times the amount of fluid lost; so for every 1 kg they should drink 1.5 litres of fluid. Alternatively, consuming 1 ml of water for every 1 calorie consumed has been shown to meet the hydration needs of children. Therefore, using the data in table 1.1 in chapter 1, a very active 9-13 year old male would require 2000-2600 kcal and subsequently 2-2.6 litres of water per day.

Urine Specific Gravity

A more accurate way to determine hydration status is to use a piece of equipment known as a refractometer and measure something called urine specific gravity (USG). Urine specific gravity compares the density of urine with the density of water. Athletes simply provide a small sample of urine and a few drops are placed on the refractometer. This then provides a number which corresponds to hydration status. Specific USG values can be found in table 4.1.

Table 4.1 Urine specific gravity (USG) and hydration status.

Hydration status	USG level
Well hydrated	<1.010
Minimal dehydration	1.010-1.020
Significant dehydration	1.020-1.030
Serious Dehydration	>1.030

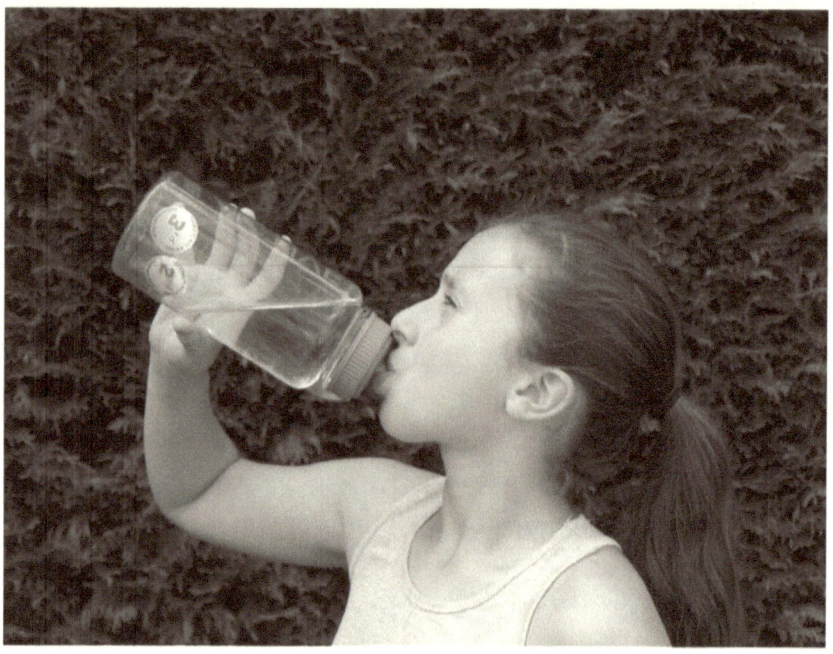

Dehydration and the Impact on Performance

Ensuring your athletes are adequately hydrated is crucial, as dehydration has been shown to negatively affect performance.[6] Whilst there is some debate as to the exact level of dehydration that leads to a decrease in performance, numerous studies have shown a decrease in body fluids of just 2-3 % can have a negative effect.[6] However, it is not only physical fitness that is decreased, as dehydration also impacts on cognitive performance, mood state and reaction time. Table 4.2 outlines the impact of different levels of dehydration on the body, while table 4.3 provides and overview of the symptoms of dehydration.

Table 4.2 Effects of dehydration level on the body.

Percent body mass lost	Physiological effects
2 %	Impaired performance & thermoregulation
4 %	Decreased muscular endurance
5 %	Heat cramps & decreased strength and endurance
7 %	Hallucinations & heat exhaustion
10 %	Circulatory collapse, heat stroke, coma & death

Table 4.3 Signs and symptoms of dehydration.

Signs of dehydration	
Dizziness	Dark urine
Light-headedness	Infrequent urination
Nausea	Dry mouth and throat
Headache	High body temperature
Muscle cramps	

Can You Have Too Much Water?

Yes, it is possible to consume too much fluid, which can lead to a condition known as hyponatremia, which is an abnormally low sodium level in the blood. However, hyponatremia under normal conditions is rare and is generally only seen in ultra-endurance events where excess fluids are consumed over several hours. If your child is continually going to the toilet and has very clear urine they may need to reduce their fluid intake, particularly close to bedtime to avoid interrupted sleep.

How to Stay Hydrated

Before Exercise

Your athlete should start the hydration process early by consuming liquids throughout the day before getting to training or competition. School children should be encouraged to take water to school with them so that they are adequately hydrated by the time they get to training or competition.

Ensure you get your child to drink fluids when eating, as this will optimise hydration due to the electrolytes in the foods, thereby aiding the retention of water and transferring it to the muscles.

Around 2 hours prior to exercise your young athlete should aim to consume between 400-600 ml of plain water. This allows time for the fluids to be adsorbed fully from the gut. Fizzy soft drinks should be avoided before exercise, as they are digested more slowly than water and can result in bloating.

During Exercise

Make sure your athlete has a water bottle at training and encourage them to take regular sips throughout training and competition. This should be roughly 150-300 ml of fluids every 15-20 minutes. Coaches should allow time between sets for children to take on fluids. If this opportunity is provided and bottles are to hand, then most children will automatically drink. Adopting this strategy during training will promote good hydration skills and more likely promote regular drinking during competition too.

However, some young athletes remain reluctant to drink during exercise. Encouraging them and providing adequate opportunity to rehydrate is probably the best way to overcome this problem until they get into the habit of keeping themselves adequately hydrated. Additionally, whilst there is evidence in adults that drinking to thirst is the best hydration strategy, encourage children to start drinking before they feel thirsty may be more beneficial, as they are not as aware of their fluid needs and may forget to drink if left to wait until thirsty, as by then they will already be starting to dehydrate and may experience a decline in performance. Remind them that elite athletes also need to drink frequently during training and competition and will always have their drinks bottle handy.

Swimmers often worry about getting a 'stitch'. While it is still not fully understood why they occur, it is thought that it may be due to the stomach wall becoming distended from food or fluid consumption immediately before or during exercise and therefore irritating the nerves and muscles in the abdomen. It is therefore advised to drink small amounts but regularly and in advance of competition. Your child should also try to avoid very sugary or carbonated fluids before training and competition to reduce distension of the stomach.

For exercise that lasts less than 60 minutes, water alone is sufficient for hydration as the body has enough energy stores to fuel exercise of this duration. Additionally, your child will not burn enough calories during 60 minutes or less to warrant a sports drink. For exercise durations longer than 60 minutes or in hot and humid conditions, a sports drink with a 6 % carbohydrate solution is beneficial to top up fluid levels and to maintain energy. These drinks should also contain some sodium, as this will help with the adsorption of the fluids. Again, your child should aim to sip 150-300 ml every 15-20 minutes.

Post Exercise

The focus of post exercise hydration is to return the muscles to their pre-exercise state. Within the first 30 minutes after your child's session, encourage them to rest and have a larger drink. This could be something like a specific sports recovery drink, though plain milk or flavoured milkshakes are just as effective as expensive sports recovery drinks. Following the first 30 minutes, fluid intake should be as desired during the few hours post exercise, though remember that fluid intake post exercise should be 1.5 times the fluids lost during exercise. Rehydration should also be combined with appropriate food intake.

Do Children Need Sports Drinks?

On a day to day basis, there should be no need for children to consume sports/energy drinks. Sports drinks frequently contain significant amount of sugar and caffeine and as a result, frequent long term use may negatively impact on the dental health and weight management of the child. With forward planning and preparation, children should be able to get the energy required for training and competition through real foods, whilst water should be the preferred fluid of choice to maintain hydration, unless exercise is of an extended duration as outlined above. In an ideal world, all young athletes would drink only water and healthy fluids. However, at the end of the day, your young athlete is still a child and the occasional sugary drink post exercise as a treat is fine, as long as it doesn't become the norm.

References

1. Falk, B. and Dotan, R. (2008) Children's thermoregulation during exercise in the heat – a revisit. *Applied Physiology, Nutrition and Metabolism*, 33(2), 420-427.
2. Rowland, T. (2008) Thermoregulation during exercise in the heat in children: old concepts revisited. *Journal of Applied Physiology*, https://doi.org/10.1152/japplphysiol.01196.2007.
3. Kawahata, A. (1960) Sex differences in sweating. In: *Essential Problems in Climatic Physiology*, edited by Yoshimura, H., Ogata, K. and Kyoto, S., Japan, Nankodo, p.169-184.
4. Rees, J. and Shuster, S. Pubertal induction of sweat gland activity. *Clinical Science* (London), 60, 689-692.
5. Austin, K. and Seebohar, B. (2011) Performance Nutrition: Applying the science of nutrient timing, *Human Kinetics*, Champaign, IL, 80-81.
6. Cheuvront, SN., Carter, R. and Sawka, MN. (2003) Fluid balance and endurance exercise performance. *Current Sports Medicine Reports*, 2(4), 202-208.

CHAPTER 5: WEIGHT MANAGEMENT

Parents and coaches will often worry over whether their child/athlete is a healthy weight. However, it is important to remember children, like adults, come in all shapes and sizes and while some will inevitably struggle to keep weight down, others may find it hard to consume enough calories to put weight on. This can be frustrating for the child and worrying for the parents and coaches. Whilst there is often a linear relationship between body weight and exercise performance, this relationship doesn't always hold true for young athletes. Therefore, it is imperative that parents and coaches do not make it a big issue about body weight, as insensitive handling of such issues may result in the child developing an unhealthy relationship with food and body image.

Whilst it may seem a logical approach to monitor the food intake of your child, overtly counting calories in front of your child can lead to disordered eating[1], though this may only be triggered several months or even years later. Keep in mind that girls around the age of 9 to 10 and boys 10 to 11 will start puberty and naturally lay down more fat. Therefore, it is recommended that parents and coaches try to promote healthy eating habits, as this has been shown to lead to long term health and wellbeing when done when children are young.

Weight Gain and Exercise Performance

Weight gain can be both desirable (through increased lean muscle mass) and undesirable (through increases in fat mass). Being larger and stronger can be advantageous for sports such as rugby, football and basketball, whilst for some sports that may be weight categorised such as boxing or judo, or artistic sports such as gymnastics, being strong without weight gain may be more appropriate. It is important to bear in mind though, that while for most sports leanness generally leads to improved performance, being excessively lean and excessively overweight can both compromise health and performance. There is also no single optimal body weight and lean muscle mass for all individuals and each child will perform best within a body weight range specific to them. However, if your young athlete is genuinely overweight, then any weight loss programme should be done following the advice of your doctor, nutritionist or dietician.

As alluded to above, during puberty children will naturally increase fat depositions. This increase in fat levels is particularly important for females at this age, as it influences the onset of menarche (the first menstrual cycle). Research has shown that young females of prepubescent age who exhibit lower than average body fat levels experience a delay in the onset of menarche.[2] However, one study of over 2300 girls also indicated a trend for the earlier onset of menses over the past 30 years, as a result of increase fat levels and obesity.[3] Therefore, the importance of healthy eating education at this age cannot be underestimated.

Boys will also lay down more fat at this age and will often look chubby around the midriff. Subsequently, though exercise performance may decrease during this period, structured weight loss programmes during this phase of development should not be recommended, as it may interfere with the natural growth and development of both male and female children. Parents and coaches should reassure their young athletes that this is a normal part of growing up and is a temporary phase.

Generally speaking, restrictive dieting does not work for either adults or children. This is largely because they are difficult to adhere to long term and once a particular food is forbidden the individual will tend to crave it even more, reducing the likelihood of them sticking to the diet plan. Instead, children should be educated on healthy eating and portion sizes and encouraged to make small modifications to their eating and drinking habits that they are more likely to stick to in the long run.

As a parent or coach of a child that *is* overweight, it is important that you refrain from discussing the issue publicly and not to compare the child's body weight and subsequent performance to that of other children. There are however some tips you can use to promote better eating habits. These are outlined in table 5.1.

Table 5.1 Recommendations for preventing weight gain.

Tip	Reason why
Don't skip meals & include snacks	Frequent meal skipping can lead children to 'graze' more, which often leads to overconsumption of calories, more so than a proper meal. Having scheduled meal times and including healthy snacks can help avoid such grazing and subsequently control hunger and weight.
Slow down when eating	Children often rush their food, which leads to poor digestion and overeating due to not feeling full. Getting your child to slow down and chew food more fully can help address these two issues.
Plate up before sitting down	If people are given the opportunity to plate up their own food from serving bowls on the table, they are more likely to over eat (think '*all you can eat*' buffet cart). Therefore, always put your child's food on a plate for them and keep serving dishes off the table.
Avoid drinking calories	Drinks are an easy way to get calories in quickly without affecting appetite. This means it is also too easy to over-consume calories. Drinking 200 kcals will not satisfy hunger as much as eating 200 kcals. Therefore, where possible your child should eat their calories and drink simply to hydrate.
Wait 20 minutes	Rather than your child helping themselves to a second serving after a meal, make them wait 20 minutes to allow the meal to start digesting. This will often lead them to not needing the extra portion anymore.

In addition to the tips in table 5.1 parents should try to get children who are overweight to move more outside of structured exercise sessions. This could be as simple as encouraging them to walk or cycle to school or heading out on a family walk. Parents should also refrain from allowing children to snack while watching television, as it is easy to lose track of what is being consumed. Also, whilst stated previously in this book that low fat options should not be the norm for children, for those that are overweight, substituting full fat dairy for low fat options may be a suitable recommendation, though again beware of added sugars.

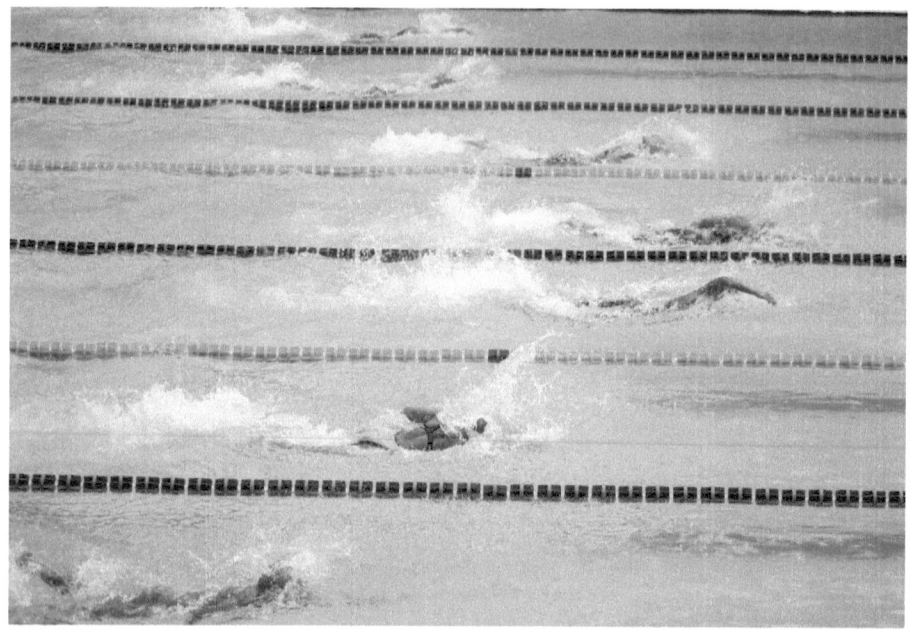

Weight Loss and Exercise Performance

While some young athletes may struggle with weight loss, others may find it equally difficult to gain weight. For activities such as football, rugby, hockey etc. being bigger can be a distinct advantage. Very active and particularly slim, lean children may find it hard to increase muscle mass to enable them to compete on an equal level with their larger peers. However, as previously discussed, children grow at different rates and being thin doesn't always mean they are unhealthy. Likewise, underweight children tend to catch up to their earlier developing peers by their late teens, meaning weight gain strategies are generally not necessary.

Some children can be underweight or very thin as a result of illness or eating disorders. Chapter 7 covers some of the more common eating disorders and what signs and symptoms to look out for, though it is important that parents and coaches address suspected cases with sensitivity and seek professional advice.

For healthy children who do need to increase weight, any intervention should only be introduced after puberty once the child has matured and a better idea of what weight gain is needed can be established. If weight gain is required, then the following tips can be used to help young athletes increase muscle mass.

Table 5.2 Recommendations for increasing lean body weight.

Tip	Reason why
Create a positive energy balance	In order to increase body/muscle mass, a positive energy balance needs to be created. This means eating more energy than the energy they burn. However, this can mean a significant increase in calories as a result of increased exercise intensity. An increase of 300-500 kcals per day is recommend to promote steady weight gain.
More regular eating	Assuming your athlete needs 3000 kcals per day, this is a lot of food to eat during a typical breakfast, lunch, dinner eating plan. Therefore, spreading food intake out over 3 main meals and 3-4 smaller, regular snacks will help prevent feeling bloated and put less burden on the athlete to each large volumes of food per sitting.
Increase protein	Protein is required for muscle growth. Therefore, it stands to reasons that increasing the child's intake will aid the process of weight gain. However, at this age protein supplements should be avoided in favour of whole foods such as lean meats and dairy.
Nutrient dense snacks	To increase overall calorie intake, aim to introduce healthy, nutrient dense snacks such as oatmeal, rice pudding, dried fruits, nuts and yogurt.

If a young athlete is struggling to meet their energy requirements or failing to gain body mass at an expected rate, then increasing the amount of healthy unsaturated fats in their diet may also help address this issue.

Assessing Body Weight

Assessing the weight of children should be done carefully, as it shouldn't be made into a big issue. However, there are some tools that can be used to assess if a child's body weight is 'healthy'.

Height-Weight Charts

Simple height-weight charts are probably the easiest means of assessing your child's body weight. Using these charts, you simply draw a horizontal line across from the child's height and a vertical line up from their weight and the intersecting point provides an indication of whether the child is a healthy weight, overweight or obese.

However, despite the simplicity of height-weight charts, they are severely limited in that they do not differentiate between fat mass and fat free mass. As such, it is possible to have a child that is very muscular and yet they will show as overweight or even obese on such charts. Therefore, these charts should be used only as a rough guide.

Body Mass Index (BMI)

Body mass index (BMI) is similar in many ways to height-weight charts, in that it provides an assessment of whether you are a healthy weight for your height. BMI is measured in kg/m^2, though rather than assessing body fat it simply reflects whole body weight.[4] BMI ranges have been developed to indicate whether someone is underweight (BMI under 18.5), healthy weight (BMI 18.6-24.9), overweight (BMI 25-29.9), obese (BMI 30-39.9) or extremely obese (BMI over 40).[5]

However, while these charts may appear more accurate as they give a specific value for BMI, like height-weight charts, BMI does not distinguish between what is fat or muscle and subsequently can also be misleading. Action should not be taken based on BMI values alone, instead you should consult your doctor or qualified nutritionist or dietician if you have any concerns. Figure 5.1 illustrates a typical BMI chart. To get a rough estimate of your child's BMI, simply find their weight and height and draw straight lines until they intersect. Where they cross the number underneath is your BMI.

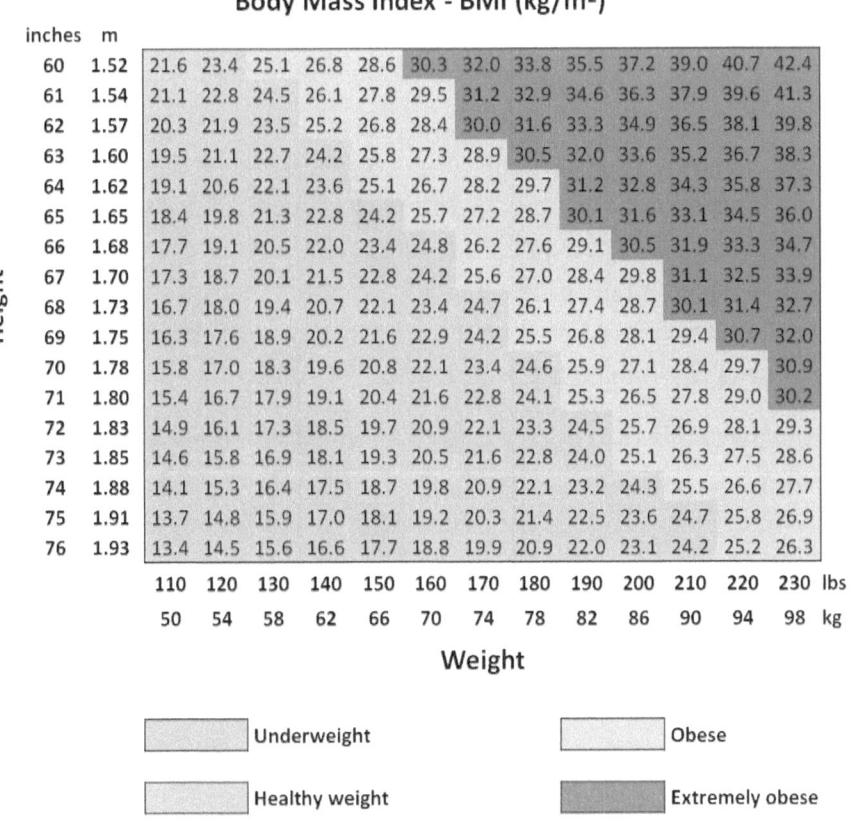

Figure 5.1. Body mass index table.

Bioelectrical Impedance Analysis

Bioelectrical impedance analysis (BIA) measures the resistance by the body to a small undetectable, painless electrical current when passed through it. It is used to estimate total body water and in turn percentage body fat. Whilst these systems are easy to use, they require strict controls in order to get accurate values. It is recommended that the individual being tested refrains from eating 4 hours prior to testing, performs no exercise within 12 hours of the test, consumes no diuretics (substances that make you urinate) within 7 days and empties the bladder 30 minutes before testing. Clearly such strict controls are difficult to enforce for adults let alone children. Therefore, this method may not be the most practical for use with young athletes.

Skinfold Measurements

Lastly, skinfold assessments involve taking several measurements at different sites on the body by pinching the skin and underlying fat between the thumb and finger and applying callipers to record the thickness of the skinfold. This technique is based on the principle that approximately half of the body's fatty tissue lies directly beneath the skin. Predictive equations are then used to estimate body fat levels.

However, this technique requires a trained anthropometrist to conduct the testing and unless the assessor has significant experience, values can be grossly under or overestimated. Despite this, skinfold assessments are becoming more commonly used in youth teams and do provide the most accurate measure assuming they are performed by skilled personnel.

Exercise and Eating Disorders

Eating disorders are serious mental illnesses and the Academy for Eating Disorders states that they warrant the same levels of medical care as other mental health illnesses, such as depression and bipolar disorder.[6] Those with eating disorders and those with disordered eating often exhibit many of the same traits such as an unhealthy relationship with food or certain food groups, body weight and body image. While it can be difficult to determine whether someone has disordered eating patterns or a full blown eating disorder, the differences generally lie in the frequency and level of obsession with eating behaviours and the distress this causes the individual. However, clinical diagnosis of an eating disorder is established using criteria set out by the Diagnostic and Statistical Manual of Mental Disorders, version 4 (DSM-IV).

While some people may legitimately avoid consuming certain foods due to medical conditions (for example those with celiac disease cannot eat gluten containing foods), disordered eating has become more mainstream over the past decade due to the promotion of popular fad diets, such as veganism, paleo and gluten free diets. Subsequently, due to the increased social acceptability of these diets, it has made the diagnosis of genuine illnesses more difficult. Disordered eating has also been exacerbated by the introduction of terms like 'clean eating' whereby particular foods are demonised and perceived as bad for us. As such, those with disordered eating are more susceptible to developing full blown eating disorders.

With respect to exercise, successful athletes can be described as driven, perfectionist, obsessive, high achieving and competitive. Unfortunately, these are also the same traits presented by those with eating disorders. Subsequently, research has shown that young athletic children may be more at risk of developing disordered eating and eating disorders than their less active peers, resulting from engaging in a culture obsessed with appearance and the knowledge of how food can influence performance.[7,8,9] Thankfully though, despite their understanding of foods role in performance, not all young athletes will develop an unhealthy relationship with food. However, as parents and coaches it is important to be able to identify the warning signs of these conditions and to understand their effects on health as well as exercise performance.

Signs and Symptoms of Eating Disorders

The signs and symptoms of eating disorders can be a combination of behavioural, physical and psychological signs. If you suspect one of your athletes may be exhibiting several signs of an eating disorder, it is important to seek professional advice as soon as possible, as early intervention has been shown to promote recovery. It is also important to understand that the warning signs may not be easy to spot, as individuals with eating disorders may not realise that they have a problem or may try to hide the signs and symptoms due to feeling of shame and guilt. Below is an overview of some to the signs to look out for, but is by no means a comprehensive list.

Behavioural Signs

- Constant counting calories, skipping meals, fasting, avoidance of certain food or food groups
- Evidence of binge eating
- Evidence of vomiting or laxative abuse (e.g. frequent trips to the bathroom during or shortly after meals)
- Excessive exercise patterns (e.g. even when injured, refusal to stop exercising for any reason, exhibiting distress if unable to exercise)
- Making lists of 'good' and 'bad' foods
- Development of patterns or obsessive rituals around food preparation and eating
- Avoidance of all social situations involving food
- Obsessive interest in body shape and weight
- Repetitive use of weighing scales
- Social withdrawal or isolation from friends
- Deceptive behaviour such as secretly throwing out food, eating in secret or lying about the amount or type of food eaten
- Denial of hunger

Physical Signs

- Unexplained decrease in exercise performance
- Significant or rapid weight loss
- Frequent changes in weight
- Sensitivity to the cold (feeling cold most of the time, even in warm conditions)
- Loss or disturbance of menstrual periods (females)
- Signs of frequent vomiting - swollen cheeks/jawline, calluses on knuckles, or damage to teeth
- Fainting or dizziness
- Excessive and constant fatigue

Psychological Signs

- Fear of weight gain
- Preoccupation with food or with activities relating to food
- Extreme negative body image (e.g. complaining they look/feel fat when actually a healthy weight or even underweight)
- Very sensitive to comments about body, eating or exercise habits
- Increased anxiety, particularly around meal times
- Depression
- Mood swings and/or irritability
- Low self-esteem

Types of Eating Disorders

According to the Diagnostic and Statistical Manual of Mental Disorders, there are four recognised and diagnosable eating disorders. The most commonly known are anorexia nervosa and bulimia nervosa, with the others being binge-eating disorder and anorexia athletica.

Anorexia Nervosa

A diagnosis of anorexia nervosa is made when a person:

- Weighs 15 % lower than the minimum average for height
- Has an intense fear of weight gain
- Is preoccupied with food
- Socially withdraws
- Has low self-esteem
- Has distorted perception of body image
- Has a loss of menstrual period (females)
- Exercises excessively

Bulimia Nervosa

Is defined as the uncontrolled consumption of excessive amount of food followed by purging to get rid of it. Purging include vomiting, laxative use or excessive exercising. Symptoms of bulimia nervosa include:

- Excessive food consumption and purging
- Weight fluctuations, though generally a 'normal' weight
- Depression and mood swings
- Making excuses to go to the bathroom following a meal
- Dental problems
- Digestive issues such as diarrhoea, constipation and bloating
- Low self-esteem

Anorexia Athletica

A diagnosis of anorexia athletica is often used with athletes who do not meet all the criteria for a diagnosis of other eating disorders, but do exhibit signs of disordered eating patterns. Indicators of anorexia athletics include:

- Restrictive eating
- Compulsive exercising
- Amenorrhea - one or more missed menstrual periods
- Fear of getting fat
- Episodes of binge-eating

Binge-Eating Disorder

Defined as reoccurring binge-eating, but without the compulsion to purge afterwards. Signs of binge-eating disorder include:

- Digestive problems
- Fast feeding
- Weight gain
- Dieting without weight loss
- 'Normal' eating socially, but binge-eating when alone

- Emotional eating
- Feelings of guilt following a binge

Along with getting professional help, if you suspect your child has an eating disorder it is important that you consider what and how you are going to approach the situation in advance of sitting down with them. Don't try to present 'evidence' but simply state your concerns in a tactful manner, but expect them to deny it at first. Also, do not try to give advice yourself, as they require trained medical personnel to deal with it. Lastly, many young athletes will not be forthcoming about such conditions for fear of losing their place on the team. Therefore, reassure them that disclosing their problems will not affect their positon within the team in any way.

The Female Athlete Triad

The female athlete triad is the interrelationship of menstrual dysfunction, low energy availability (with or without disordered eating or an eating disorder) and reduced bone mineral density, and is relatively common in young athletic women.[10] As discussed earlier in this chapter, many young athletes feel pressured to conform to a certain body image and as such are at an increased risk of developing eating disorders or adopt disordered eating patterns. This is particularly concerning for young female athletes, as excessive exercise, under eating or a combination of both can lead to low energy availability. In less serious cases this may lead to irregular periods and decreased performance, whilst in more serious cases menstruation may cease completely for prolonged periods of time and bone mineral losses may contribute to the development of osteoporosis and stress fractures. Parents and coaches should monitor their young female athletes for signs of fatigue, weight loss, signs of stress fractures and changes in eating habits.

Treatment for the female athlete triad is relatively easy in some respects, as normal menstruation and low energy availability can be resolved through reducing training loads and ensuring the athlete gets plenty of rest combined with a balanced diet containing sufficient calcium and vitamin D. However, the nutritional aspect of the triad is often the most complex to address, as frequently this is linked to disordered eating. Therefore, a multidisciplinary approach involving doctors, coaches, nutritionists and parents may be needed. As discussed previously for eating disorders, it is important parents and coaches do not try to resolve issues related to the female athlete triad themselves, and instead seek professional advice as soon as possible.

Injury and Nutrition

Unfortunately, injury is an inevitable consequence of regular athletic training and performance, and most athletes will succumb to some form of injury at some point, whether minor or serious. These injuries can present a challenging time for athletes of all ages due to enforced rest, reduced or no training, concerns about weight gain and muscle loss etc. Therefore, managing their nutritional requirements during this period is crucial in order to aid recover and possibly help prevent injury reoccurring.

Though many injuries may result in time away from exercise, large reductions in calorie intake may not be necessary to prevent unwanted weight gain as recovery is an energy intensive process, particularly with respect to broken bones. With respect to bone fractures and breaks, energy intake can be as high as 6000 kcals per day depending on the severity of the injury. Studies have shown that energy intake can be increased as much as 20 % above resting levels during many injuries.[11]

Whilst your athlete may need to consume less energy than when performing regular exercise, due to the energy demands of the recovery process, calorie intake will generally still be greater than when not exercising. Any calories that are cut from the diet should not be from protein sources, as these are important to the healing process.

There are two main stages to exercise-induced injuries, the first being the immobilization/atrophy (muscle loss) stage and the second the return of mobility stages. The duration of the immobilization stage will largely depend upon the type and severity of the injury, but can last from as little as a few days to several month and can lead to muscle loss and reductions in strength and functionality due to disuse.[12] During the return to mobility stage, rehabilitation occurs and there is a gradual increase in physical activity again and a subsequent recovery in muscle mass. Nutrition can play a key role in each of these stages. However, parents, coaches and athletes should bear in mind that full restoration of muscle mass takes significantly longer than the time it takes to lose it.[11] Therefore, don't expect your child to return to pre-injury fitness and strength levels too soon.

Within the immobilization stage there are also several 'phases', these being the inflammation, proliferation and remodelling phases. The inflammation phase starts immediately following an injury and is characterised by pain, swelling, redness and heat around the injury site. Whilst this phase can be very uncomfortable for the athlete, inflammation is necessary to kick start tissue/bone repair and trying to completely eliminate it can be counterproductive to the healing process. However, inflammation should still be managed, as an excess can also compromise recovery. Therefore, during this initial phase, athletes should increase their intake of anti-inflammatory foods including fish oils and fish, such as salmon and mackerel, avocados, olive oil, nuts and seeds, whilst reducing intake of pro-inflammatory foods such as vegetable oils, highly processed foods and foods that contain saturated and trans fats.

The proliferation phase is primarily associated with removal of damaged tissue and deposition of new collagen fibres and the formation of scar tissue. Additionally, new blood supplies to the injured site are developed, followed finally by a reduction in the size of the wound site. During this phase and as a result of immobilization, protein balance, i.e. the balance between protein production and protein break down, shifts to a negative balance, as less protein is synthesised, while at the same time muscle proteins are broken down. Therefore, it makes sense that protein intake should increase during this period to offset any losses. Despite this suggestion though, limited research exists on humans showing that protein can adequately address muscle protein losses during injury due to a process known as 'anabolic resistance'. Anabolic resistance describes the reduced stimulation of muscle protein production to a given dose of ingested protein and contributes to declines in skeletal muscle mass. However, there *is* some evidence to suggest that the amino acid leucine has the potential to overcome anabolic resistance and help maintain muscle mass.[13]

While muscle and tendon protein losses may not respond significantly to increased protein supplementation, bone fractures do appear to benefit.[14] Therefore, it is suggested that young athletes at least maintain protein intake or increase it slightly during periods of exercise-induced immobility and ensure they prioritise protein sources that contain high levels of leucine, such as cheese, soybeans, beef, chicken, pork, nuts, seeds, fish, seafood, and beans. Though limited research exists on leucine requirements for healthy children, one study suggested this should be approximately 44 mg/kg body mass per day. This is around 10 % higher than recommendations for adults.[15] Therefore, a 60 kg child would require 2640 mg leucine per day. As a guide per 100 g of each, lean chicken breast contains around 2652 mg leucine, tuna steak around 2431 mg, eggs 1075 mg, tofu 3644 mg, soybeans 2868 mg and ricotta cheese around 1235 mg of leucine.

Finally, there is the 'remodelling' phase, where the scar tissue developed during the initial phases is broken down and replaced by a stronger form of collagen to complete the healing process. Nutritional considerations during this phase are similar to those of the proliferation phase. Figure 5.2 summarises the nutritional considerations when dealing with injuries and bone fractures.

Calorie Intake	Calcium Intake	Protein Intake	Vitamins and Minerals
Though activity may be reduced, injuries (particularly fractures) require a large number of kcals to heal effectively. This can be as much as 6000 kcals per day depending upon the severity and the individual. Any calorie restriction should not come from protein.	Adequate calcium intake is essential for bone remodelling. Aim for ~1500 mg/day from sources such as cheese, yogurt, collard greens, kale, broccoli and almonds.	Protein is needed for development of new bone and muscle tissue, skeletal integrity and immune response. Protein intake of 15-20 g/day have been shown to aid fracture healing. Include poultry lean meat, eggs, nuts and legumes.	Increasing intake of iron (~15-18 mg), zinc and vitamins A,D,E,K and C will help boost haemoglobin production, thus oxygen supply, calcium absorption and antioxidant content. Include oily fish, fruit, vegetables, eggs and fortified milk in your diet.

Figure 5.2 Nutritional considerations for injury.

References

1. Scaglioni, S., Salioni, M. and Galimberti, C. (2008) Influence of parental attitudes in the development of children eating behaviour. *British Journal of Nutrition*, 99(1), S22-S25.
2. Kaplowitz, PB. (2008) Link between body fat and the timing of puberty. *Pediatrics*, 121, S208.

3. Biro, FM., McMahahon, RP., Striegel-Moore, R. et al. (2001) Impact of timing of pubertal maturation on growth in black and white female adolescents: The National Heart, Lung and Blood Institute Growth and Health Study. *Journal of Pediatrics*, 138(5), 636-643.

4. Freedman, DS. and Sherry, B. (2009) The validity of BMI as an indicator of body fatness and risk among children. *Pediatrics*, 124(1), S23-S34.

5. Gallagher, D., Heymsfield, SB., Heo, M., Jebb, SA., Murgatroyd, PR. and Sakamoto, Y. (2000) Healthy percentage body fat ranges: an approach for developing guidelines based on body mass index. *The American Journal of Clinical Nutrition*, 72(3), 694-701.

6. Klump, KL., Bulik, CM., Kaye, WH., Treasure, J. and Tyson, E. (2008) Academy for eating disorders position paper: Eating disorders are serious mental illnesses. *International Journal of Eating Disorders*, 42(2), 97-103.

7. Davis, C., Katzman, D., Kaptein, S., Kirsh, C., Brewer, H., Kalmbach, K. et al., (1997) The prevalence of high-level exercise in the eating disorders: Etiological implications. *Comprehensive Psychiatry*, 38(6), 321-326.

8. Picard, CL. (1999) The level of competition as a factor for the development of eating disorders in female collegiate athletes. *Journal of Youth and Adolescence*, 28(5), 583-594.

9. Martinsen, M., Bahr, R., Borresen, R., Holme, I., Pensgaard, AM. and Sundgot-Borgen, J. (2014) Preventing eating disorders among young elite athletes: A randomised controlled trial. *Medicine and Science in Sports and Exercise*, 46(3), 435-447.

10. Nazem, TG. and Ackerman, KE. (2012) The female athlete triad. *Sports Health*, 4(4), 302-311.

11. Frankenfield, D. (2006) Energy expenditure and protein requirements after traumatic injury. *Nutrition in Clinical Practice*, 21, 430-437.

12. Jones, SW., Hill, RJ., Krasney, PA., O'Conner, B., Peirce, N. and Greenhaff, PL. (2004) Disuse atrophy and exercise rehabilitation in humans profoundly affects the expression of genes associated with the regulation of skeletal muscle mass. *FASEB J*, 18, 1025-1027.

13. Rieu, I. (2006) Leucine supplementation improves muscle protein synthesis in elderly men independently of hyperaminoacidemia. *Journal of Physiology*, 575, 305-315.
14. Eneroth, M., Olsson, UB. and Thorngren, KG. (2006) Nutritional supplementation decreases hip fracture-related complications. *Clinical Orthopaedics and Related Research*, 451, 212-217.
15. Mager, DR., Wykes, LJ., Ball, RO. and Pencharz, PB. (2003) Branched-chain amino acid requirements in school-aged children determined by indicator amino acid oxidation (IAAO). *The Journal of Nutrition*, 133(11), 3540-3545.

CHAPTER 6: SUPPLEMENTS

When compared to other sciences, nutritional science is still relatively new. Major advances in our understanding of the impact nutrition makes to health and performance have only coming in the past 20-30 years. However, there is still much confusing 'evidence' about what we should and shouldn't consume, which seems to change year on year.

This is especially true for active/athletic populations. When considering youth athletes, their nutritional requirements lie heavily on the growing phases of puberty and adolescence in addition to providing fuel for increased physical activity. This is where the nutrition supplement industry appears to have a jump start on academics and nutritionists. We live in an age where people wants a 'quick fix' and supplement companies claim to know what we need to jump higher, run faster, bulk up or get slimmer quicker.

Breaking news!! Most of these supplements have little scientific evidence to support their manufacturers' claims. Ron Maughan, Professor of Sports Nutrition and Chair of the International Olympic Committee's (IOC) Medical Commission's Sports Nutrition Group, once stated in relation to supplements *"If it works, then it's probably banned, if it's not banned, then it probably doesn't work!"*. However, whilst there are some notable exceptions, such as caffeine, carbohydrate, protein and β-alanine, on the whole Prof Maughan did have a valid point.

Supplement companies often take nutritional concepts that should work (in theory) and use these to promote their products. However, the reality is that these concepts often either haven't been proven yet (at least in human experiments), or the proposed metabolic/biochemical pathways involved are much more complicated in practice and involve numerous supplement/supplement interactions or supplement/drug interactions etc.

Subsequently, very few supplements should be recommended for children under the age of 16 years without appropriate supervision. If parents implement a well-balanced and nutritious diet there should be no need to include supplements. However, parents and coaches should be mindful that young athletes are often inquisitive about supplements, especially when they see adult athletes taking them and their heroes endorsing them. Despite this, this doesn't mean supplements are always safe for children to take. Therefore, it is useful for you as a parents and/or coach to be knowledgeable about the benefits and risks of supplementation in order to educate your young athletes.

It would be somewhat naive to pretending sports supplements are un-common or don't exist in youth sport. They do, and this is unlikely to change any time soon. The dietary supplement sector in the US was worth $115 billion in 2018 and is projected to grow a further 8 % by 2025. Of this, sports nutrition accounted for approximately $8 billion.[1] With reference to the scale of supplement usage in youth, one study reported between 24-29 % of youths had taken performance enhancing supplements[2], the National Health Interview Survey in the US reported that 94 % of teens regularly used vitamin supplements[3], whilst in the UK 62 % of youth track and field athletes reported taking sports supplements.[4]

Supplements Vs. Ergogenic Aids

Supplements

The terms '*supplements*' and '*ergogenic aids*' are often used inter-changeably, yet there are important differences. As their name suggests, di-etary supplements are any products intended for oral ingestion to supple-ment the diet and they must contain one or more of the following ingredi-ents: vitamins, minerals, herbs or botanicals, amino acids, enzymes, organ tissues or metabolites. Dietary supplements are intended for ingestion in ei-ther pill, capsule or liquid form, must not be represented as a conventional food or a sole item or meal and must be clearly labelled as a 'dietary sup-plement'.

In the US, dietary supplements are 'regulated' (and I use the term 'regulated' loosely) under the umbrella of 'foods' by the Food and Drug Administration (FDA) and the Dietary Supplement Health and Education Act of 1994 (DSHEA), whilst the advertising of such products is governed by the Federal Trade Commission (FTC). Similarly, in the UK supplements are regulated by the Food Standards Agency (FSA) under the Food Safety Act 1990.

Despite this apparent regulation, there are numerous loopholes within these legislations that allow for spurious claim of effectiveness without proof and there is no formal requirement for review or approval by the FDA or FSA. As a result of this rather lax control, it has created a 'buyer beware' market. As long as a supplement does not claim to 'cure', advertising can be somewhat misleading (just look at diet pills, there is little evidence they work despite manufacturers claims).

Ingredient content and quality can also be an issue with dietary supplements. Any supplement approved by the FDA prior to 1994 can subsequently change the ingredients without further approval, unless that ingredient did not exist prior to 1994. Once on sale to the public, it is the manufacturers' responsibility to ensure the product is safe. It is only if there are suspicions that a supplement is ineffective, unsafe that the FDA will then try to remove it from sale. However, as there is no requirement for manufacturers to investigate potential problem cases, the FDA relies heavily on consumers to report issues themselves.

The issue of supplement ingredients is a particular problem for athletes and due to the loose regulatory controls it is not uncommon for supplements to become contaminated. Research by Green et al[5] examined the ingredients of 12 different over the counter steroids and reported the following observations:

- 11/12 contained less than 90 % or more than 110 % of the ingredient amounts listed on label.
- 5/12 contained at least one ingredient not listed on label.
- 2/12 were missing at least one ingredient listed on label.

- One brand contained 10 mg of testosterone, a controlled steroid.

In a similar study, Geyer et al[6] investigated 634 commonly used supplements and found that 14.8 % contained steroids not listed on label. These studies show how easy it would be to ingest a banned substance unknowingly. However, despite this the World Anti-Doping Agency (WADA) and UK Anti-Doping (UKAD) enforce a policy of 'strict liability'. In other words, it is ultimately the athletes' responsibility to ensure the supplements or foods they consume are safe and banned substance free. Claims of inadvertent doping are not accepted justification by these organisations. As a UK Anti-Doping Advisor, I have a responsibility for educating athletes and support personnel on what supplements are safe or not and the merits of those supplements for enhancing performance. Generally, I will always adopt a food first approach and only suggest supplements if absolutely necessary.

As a parent and/or coach it is important for you to be aware that there are 10 Anti-Doping Rule Violations (ADRVs). All 10 apply to athletes and six (in bold) also apply to athlete support personnel, i.e. you. Therefore, you can be sanctioned along with the athlete.

Anti-Doping Rule Violations (ADRVs)

1. Presence
2. Use
3. Evading, refusing
4. Whereabouts failures
5. Tampering or attempted tampering
6. Possession
7. Trafficking or attempted trafficking
8. Administration, aiding, abetting
9. Complicity
10. Prohibited Association

If you wish to learn more about these rules, please visit the UK Anti-Doping website (www.ukad.org.uk/anti-doping-rules) or visit the World

Anti-Doping Agency (WADA) website (www.wada-ama.org/en). Ultimately, what these rules means for you, is that you are also responsible for any drug violations caused by contaminated supplements or otherwise. Another useful resource is the Global Drug Reference Online (www.Global-DRO.com) website. Whilst this doesn't contain information that applies to dietary supplements, it does provide information on the prohibited status of specific medications based on the current WADA prohibited list. This is a searchable database where athletes and support personnel can check if a particular medication/ingredient is on the prohibited list or not or whether there is an accepted upper limit.

Ergogenic Aids

Unlike dietary supplements, ergogenic aids are supplements specifically marketed to enhance performance that is generally sports related. They are also regulated by the FDA and FSA in the US and UK respectively, but unlike dietary supplements, it is the FDA/FSA that must prove the product is safe or not, rather than the manufacturer.

Enhancing sport and/or exercise performance may relate to improving recovery from exercise, enhancing weight loss or gain, or giving you more energy. These claims are similar to those of many dietary supplements, therefore manufacturers will often seek to classify ergogenic aids as a supplement instead due to the less stringent regulations imposed on dietary supplements.

As stated previously, I am generally against recommending sports supplements for children (with the exception of carbohydrate drinks for prolonged training sessions). However, if your child *is* going to supplement then it is advised they look for sports supplements with the following logos on the labelling, as the 'Informed-Sport' logo ensures all batches are tests for safety and non-contamination prior to sale, whilst the 'Informed-Choice' logo ensures monthly blind sampling takes place with the market place:

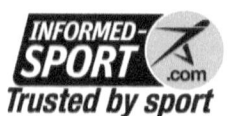 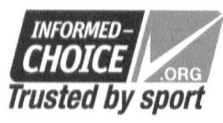

As mentioned at the start of this chapter, there is limited evidence to support the use of many/most supplements and ergogenic aids. Research into the effectiveness of these products takes time to conduct and often manufacturers base their claims on studies performed on animals rather than humans. There are also many other factors to consider, such as the participants used in the study, i.e. where they elite athletes or recreational exercises? Why should we expect the responses to a particular product be the same for both groups, as physiologically they are very different and the higher dosages often used by elite athletes have not been well studied. Additionally, elite athletes also present a very small portion of the supple-ment/ergogenic aid market; therefore, manufacturers will most often target the general public as they provide a bigger source of income. Also, were the products they tested in a fed or fasted state and was it administered in pill, powder or liquid form? This may influence the potential potency of the product being tested.

Parents and coaches should bear the following questions in mind when discussing supplementation with their young athletes or if approached by an athlete for advice:

- Can they address the issue through diet?
- Who needs to supplement?
- Should I recommend a supplement?
- How much do they need?
- What do I recommend?
- Can they get too much?
- What scientific evidence is there to support the supplements use?

If you are unsure, seek advice from a qualified nutritionist and preferably one who is an anti-doping accredited advisor.

Commonly Used Supplements

Below I have provided an overview of some of the most common supplements used for sports performance, along with a brief discussion of their merits and risks. This is not an exhaustive list and parents/coaches should perform their own thorough research on these supplements to help educate themselves and their athletes.

Creatine

Creatine is a protein produced from amino acids naturally within the body and is also found in meat, poultry and fish in smaller quantities. It is also one of the most commonly used supplements by both adult and junior athletes, due to its well documented benefits for aiding recovery and building muscle mass. However, limited research has been conducted on children despite the prevalence of creatine use in this population (between 15-50 % of youth athletes consume creatine, depending on which journal articles you read). Of those studies that have tested creatine supplementation in youth athletes, approximately 20 g/day creatine appears beneficial for performance.[9,10] However, other studies suggest creatine uptake may be limited in children and adolescents and therefore may be of limited benefit.[11,12]

The American College of Sports Medicine (ACSM) recommend that athletes under 18 years should not use creatine and many manufacturers state this age limit on their packaging. However, as outlined in one review study[13], one should not dismiss 25+ years of research on creatine that repeatedly show it to be safe and effective in numerous populations. However, it should be noted, that those who consume a meat inclusive diet shouldn't really need to supplement with creatine, as the upper limit for creatine storage is around 160 mg, and with a meat inclusive diet people are pretty close to this already.

Caffeine

Caffeine is a stimulant drug found in coffees, teas, cola and chocolate and many sport/energy drinks. It's proposed to aid strength and speed based exercise by decreasing reaction time and increasing muscle fibre recruitment and therefore force production, whilst for endurance based sports it has been shown to decrease perception of effort, delay fatigue and increase fat metabolism. However, these responses have only been observed in adults, and limited research exists on caffeine's response in children. Due to the addictive properties of caffeine and its possible side effects, it is not recommended children consume it and while there are no guidelines in the UK, elsewhere there is a general agreement that less than 85-95 mg per day is the upper limit. As a guide, one cup of brewed coffee contains between 60 to 150 mg of caffeine, instant coffee about 100 mg, brewed tea between 20 and 50 mg, and caffeinated soft drinks about 50 mg.

Protein and Amino Acids

Protein supplements come in numerous different forms, such as pre-prepared drinks, powder, gels and bars and are used for a wide range of functions. Protein supplements contain a range of essential amino acids, including branch chain amino acids (BCAA's) such as leucine, iso-leucine and valine, which have been shown to reduce fatigue. Additionally, leucine can aid recovery, while the amino acid glutamine can help fight infection and aid health.

However, whilst generally safe for consumption by children, as discussed in chapter 2, it is not necessary for children to take protein supplements. Though active children require a higher protein intake than their non-active peers, this should be easily attained via a balanced diet that is inclusive of diary and meat, whilst vegetarian/vegan athletes can get adequate protein from sources such as black beans, nuts and seeds, tofu, quinoa, lentils etc. It is also important to remember that protein alone will not build muscle, this can only occur when adequate protein intake is combined with regular resistance based training.

Carbohydrate Sports Drinks

Carbohydrate sports drinks have been repeatedly shown to improve performance during exercise lasting longer than 1 hour.[14,15] These drinks are made up of a range of different carbohydrates such a sucrose, fructose and maltodextrin and often contain electrolytes such as sodium, potassium and magnesium, as these stimulate the thirst response making us want to drink more and therefore aid fluid retention. Typically, solutions between

4-6 %, i.e. 4-6 g carbohydrate per 100 ml water, have been shown to be absorbed quickest from the stomach.

However, it is worth considering, that despite their positive effects for exercise performance, researchers often disagree as to the potential for these sugary drinks to negatively affect dental health. There are however, a number of studies that do suggest frequent use of these drinks can lead to dental erosion. Therefore, their use with children should be limited only to prolonged (greater than 1 hour), higher intensity training sessions and competition, rather than being consumed during every session.

Additionally, most energy drinks are primarily made up of carbohydrate, but also contain high levels caffeine. Therefore, as outlined in the caffeine section above, energy drink consumption should be limited in children due to the inclusion of caffeine and the potential side effects and a greater sensitivity to these in children.

Androstenedione (Andro)

Initially developed in the 1970's in East Germany, androstenedione (Andro) it was used in nasal sprays to increase aggression shortly before performance. It is secreted naturally by the adrenal gland and gonads but also comes in supplement form and is an intermediate or precursor hormone to the production of testosterone. It is produced from the breakdown of cholesterol into dehydroepiandrosterone (DHEA) then into androstenedione. Due to the fact that it is only a short enzymatic reaction away from conversion to testosterone, it may seem logical to assume that supplementing with it increases the opportunity for more testosterone to be produced and therefore increase the potential for building more muscle mass and hence increasing performance.

On its own Andro has a very weak androgenic effect until converted into Testosterone. However, Andro can also take an alternative pathway. As alluded to previously in this book, our bodies can effectively regulate most things and if we already have enough testosterone present then Andro will generally be converted into estrogen instead, resulting in little gain in muscle mass.[7] While one study that is often used to support the marketing of Andro found blood testosterone increased following ingestion of Andro, they also saw a rapid decreased after 120 minutes. Not surprisingly though, this latter point is never mentioned $by Andro manufacturers. The study also found no changes in muscle mass, strength and body composition, again all point not used in Andro marketing.[8] This point also goes to high-light what we discussed earlier in this chapter about spurious claims by sup-plement manufacturers.

Generally, evidence to support the use of Andro is limited. One study tested it on 'untrained' males, and following 8 weeks of supplementation and weight training did report a 100 % increase in serum androstenedione levels. However, they also found a 115 % increase in serum estradiol and estrogen. Ultimately, there were no increases in strength, muscle mass or body composition.

No studies of the long term effects of Andro have yet been conducted, though side effects are thought to include early onset of puberty, growth stunting, emotional outbursts and acceleration of some cancer cell growth. Currently Andro is banned and can be detected in drug tests by the IOC, USOC, NCAA, and NFL.

β-Hydroxy-β-Methylbutyrate (Hmb)

β-Hydroxy-β-methylbutyrate (HMB) is derived from the breakdown of the BCAA leucine, where leucine is then metabolized into HMB. Our bod-ies produce around 0.2 to 0.4 g/day of HMB in the liver and muscle with 5-10 % of this coming from the breakdown of dietary leucine from foods such as catfish, avocados, citrus fruits and soy beans. Its proposed benefits in-clude increased muscle mass, strength and enhanced physical appearance, which makes in an attractive supplement for young impressionable athletes. However, HMB's benefits appear to work primarily in the early phases of a training program with lesser trained individuals.[16] In well trained and elite athletes, HMB has been shown to have very little or no effect on perfor-mance parameters, as the muscles are already well adapted to the training.[17] Whilst there are no published side effects of HMB use and it is not a banned substance, these results have only been shown in adults, as currently no research exists on the use of HMB with children, presumably due to ethical issues with supplementation within children. As HMB can be consumed in adequate amounts via diet, it is not recommended that children and young athletes take this supplement.

β-alanine

β–alanine is a non-essential amino acid, meaning the body can produce it naturally from other amino acids and therefore we don't have to rely on food intake to get this. However, small amounts can be consumed from meat, fish and poultry. It is a common ingredient in many 'pre-workout' supplements, as β–alanine aids the production of another compound, carnosine, which has been linked to improving high intensity exercise by reducing the acidity of the muscles (the burning sensation felt during very hard exercise) and therefore reducing fatigue and helping to maintain muscle force. However, limited research exists to support its use and at best what research is available is often contradictory. Some individuals have also reported paraesthesia (tingling of the skin) with high doses and it can also interfere with some cardiac medicines. Few studies have been performed on children and teens. In one study of 16 year old water polo players, 6 weeks of supplementation with 6.4 g/day β–alanine did increase ball throwing velocity, but the authors also stated it 'may also possibly' improve 200 m swimming performance, but again results were inconclusive.[18] Given the lack of credible research to support its use and the potential side effects, it is not recommended children and teens take β–alanine supplements.

As alluded to previously in this chapter, the body is very adept at processing and regulating the foods and nutrients we eat. However, many athletes often adopt the philosophy with supplements that if something works then more of it must be better. This is not the case and excess levels of supplements or other ingredients can lead to toxicity and cause damage to the liver, heart and other organs. Therefore, as a parent or coach, if you do decide a supplement is absolutely necessary, as the issue cannot be addressed via diet alone, then it is important not to exceed the recommended dose of that supplement.

References

1. Dietary Supplements Market Size Analysis Report by Ingredient (Botanicals, Vitamins), By Form, By Application (Immunity, Cardiac Health), By End User, By Distribution Channel, And Segment Forecasts, 2019 – 2025. https://www.grandviewresearch.com/industry-analysis/dietary-supplements-market

2. Lattavo, A., kopperud, A. and Rogers, PD. (2007) Creatine and other supplement. *Pediatric Clinics of North America*, 54, 765-760.

3. Evans, MW., Ndetan, H., Perko, M., Williams, R. and Walker, C. (2012) Dietary supplement use by children and adolescents in the United States to enhance sport performance: results of the National Health Interview Survey. *Journal of Primary Prevention*, 33, 3-12.

4. Nieper, A. (2005) National supplement practices in UK junior National track and field athletes. *British Journal of Sports Medicine*, 39(9), 645-649.

5. Green, GA., Catlin, DH. and Starcevic, B. (2001) Analysis of over-the-counter dietary supplements. *Clinical Journal of Sport Medicine*, 11, 254-259.

6. Geyer, H., Parr, MK., Mareck, U., Reinhart, U., Schrader, Y. and Schänzer, W. (2004) Analysis of non-hormonal nutritional supplements for anabolic-androgenic steroids – Results of an International study. *International Journal of Sports Medicine*, 25(2), 124-129.

7. King, DS., Sharp, RL., Vukovich, MD., Brown, GA., Reifenratah, TA., Uhl, NL., and Parsons, KA. (1999) Effect of oral androstenedione on serum testosterone and adaptations to resistance training in young men. *Journal of American Medical Association*, 281(21), 2020-2028.

8. Leder, BZ., Longcope, C., Catlin, DH., Ahrens, B., Schoenfeld, DA. and Finkelstein, JS. (2000) Oral androstenedione administration and serum testosterone concentrations in young men. *Journal of American Medical Association*, 282(6), 779-782.

9. Grindstaff, PD., Kreider, R., Bishop, R., Wilson, M., Wood, L., Alexander, C. et al. (1997) Effects of creatine supplementation on repetitive sprint performance and body composition in competitive swimmers. *International Journal of Sport Nutrition*, 7, 330–46.

10. Mohebbi, H., Rahnama, N., Moghadassi, M., Ranjbar, K. (2012) Effect of creatine supplementation on sprint and skill performance in Young Soccer Players. *Middle-East Journal of Science Research*, 12, 397–401.

11. Merege-Filho, CA., Otaduy, MC., de Sa-Pinto, AL., de Oliveira, MO., de Souza Goncalves, L., Hayashi, AP. et al. (2017) Does brain creatine content rely on exogenous creatine in healthy youth? a proof-of-principle study. *Applied Physiology, Nutrition and Metabolism,* 42, 128–134.

12. Solis, MY., Artioli, GG., Otaduy, MCG., Leite, CDC., Arruda, W., Veiga, RR. et al. (2017) Effect of age, diet, and tissue type on PCr response to creatine supplementation. *Journal of Applied Physiology,* 123, 407–414.

13. Kerksick, CM., Wilborn, CD., Roberts, MD., Smith-Ryan, A., Kleiner, SM., Jager, R. et al. (2018) ISSN exercise & sports nutrition review update: research & recommendations. *Journal* of the *International Society* of *Sports Nutrition*, doi: 10.1186/s12970-018-0242-y

14. Tsintzas, OK., Williams, C., Singh, R., Wilson, W. and Burrin, J. (1995) Influence of carbohydrate-electrolyte drinks on marathon running performance. *European Journal of Applied Physiology and Occupational Physiology*, 70(2), 154-160.

15. Jeukendrup, A., Brouns, F., Wagenmakers, AJM. and Saris, WHM. (1997) Carbohydrate-electrolyte feeding improves 1 h time trial cycling performance. *International Journal of Sports Medicine*, 18(2), 125-129.

16. Nissen, S., Sharp, R., Ray, M., Rathmacher, JA., Rice, J., Fuller, J. et al. (1996) The effect of the leucine metabolite β-Hydroxy-β-methylbutyrate on muscle metabolism during resistance-exercise training. Journal of Applied Physiology, 81, 2095-2104.

17. Ransone, J., Neighbors, K., Lefavi, R. and Chromiak, J. (2003) The effect of beta-hydroxy-beta-methylbutyrate on muscular strength and body composition in collegiate football players. Journal of Strength and Conditioning Research, 17(1), 34-39.
18. Claus, GM., Redvka, PE., Brisola, GMP., Malta, ES., de Araujo Bonetti de Poli, R., Miyagi, WE. And Zagatto, AM. (2017) Beta-alanine supplementation improves throwing velocities in repeated sprint ability and 200-m swimming performance in young water polo players. Pediatric Exercise Science, 29(2), 203-212.

CHAPTER 7: PUTTING IT INTO PRACTICE

S o far in this book we have focused primarily on what and how much your young athletes should be consuming to aid growth, development and performance. However, the timing of what they eat in and around training and competition is equally as important to the type of food and drink they consume, and can have a significant effect on performance and recovery. Therefore, this chapter will focus on the optimal timing of nutrition prior to, during and post training and competition. It will also provide examples of what to eat at specific time points.

Pre-Exercise Nutrition

The day before training or competition you should ensure you athletes consume adequate carbohydrates to support the energy demands of exercise. However, remember back in chapter 2 we discussed that children do not store carbohydrates as well as adults, therefore this should be a moderate increase in carbohydrates.[1] It is unnecessary to employ the practice of carbohydrate loading 24-48 hours before, as commonly done by adult athletes. Fluid intake should also be increased slightly to ensure a good state of hydration.

The focus for meals and snacks over the day should be 'fuel foods' with a reduction in high fat and high protein foods, as these promote feelings of satiety (fullness), which can lead to reduced carbohydrate intake. The evening meal the night before competition doesn't have to be complicated or fancy. Parents are often pushed for time and tired from work and other family commitments, so keep it simple and make a quick and easy pasta dish, (preferably with a non-creamy sauce) or a casserole with rice or quinoa or a stir fry with noodles. Lean burgers (not the ones from fast food outlets) with wholemeal buns and salad are also a quick, yet nutritious option. Remember to provide plenty of water to drink at this time, though some of the carbohydrates could come from fruit juice, milk or fruit smoothies, as this will reduce the burden of eating a large meal.

The day before training/competition athletes should also choose foods with a low glycemic index (see chapter 2, table 2.1), as these provide slower releasing energy and cause blood glucose levels to rise slowly.

Evening Meals Ideas

- **Pasta** - with tomato sauce, vegetables and cheese. You can add chicken, tuna or lean beef to this dish to lower the overall GI of the meal.
- **Curry** - lean chicken or vegetarian curry with chickpeas, served with steamed rice or quinoa.
- **Homemade burgers** – grill a small homemade mincemeat burger pate and top with salad on a multigrain bun.
- **Chicken wraps** - tortillas filled with roast chicken, salad and light sour cream or low fat Greek yoghurt.
- **Soup** - vegetable, lentil, chicken soup served with a crusty bread roll.
- **Homemade pizza** - pre-prepared pizza base topped with tomato passata, cherry tomatoes, mushrooms, lean ham and mozzarella (or any healthy toppings of your choice).
- **Stir-fry** – with chicken or pork and lots of vegetables. You can add in a sweet chilli or soy sauce and serve with noodles or rice.

All the above meal suggestions can easily be tweaked for vegetarian and vegan athletes.

Pre-Exercise Desserts & Snacks

• Pancakes	• Bagel with jam or honey
• Waffles	• Bananas
• Rice pudding with fruit	• Yoghurt smoothies
• Trail mix with nuts, seeds and raisins	• Canned or poached fruit (in natural juices, not syrup)
• Granola bar	• Fruit bun or fruit loaf with jam
• Fruit salad	• Rice cakes and peanut butter

Training and Competition Day Nutrition

Breakfast on the day of training/competition should again provide carbohydrates and fluid to top up stores depleted overnight. For mid-morning starts, breakfast should be eaten around two hours before to ensure the food has time to digest. A small low-fat snack can also be provided up to one hour before starting exercise to top up energy levels if your athlete becomes hungry again.

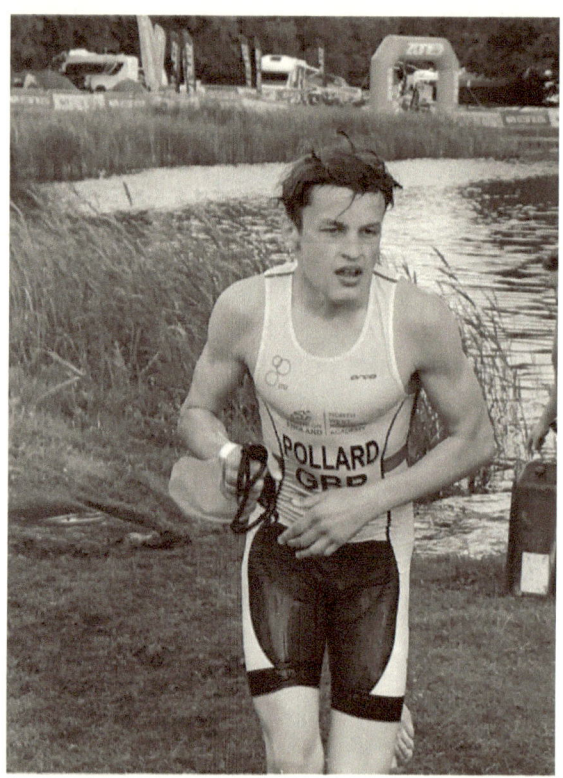

For afternoon training sessions or events, a larger breakfast should be consumed along with a pre-exercise lunch. This lunch should again be eaten approximately two hours prior to exercise starting. Evening training sessions and competitions can be a particular challenge as they are often scheduled around evening meal time. Depending on the specific time of the event, a larger afternoon snack can be given to your athlete or if later in the evening, a snack or small carbohydrate-rich dinner may be suitable a couple of hours before the event.

As a general rule aim for a 400 kcals breakfast 3-4 hours pre-exercise, or a smaller ~200 kcals snack 1.5-2 hrs pre-exercise depending of your child's training/competition schedule. 60-75 % of these calories should again be from carbohydrates. Also get your child to drink approximately 400-600 ml water with the meal or snack.

There will be occasions when the specific start time of a competition may not be known ahead of time. In these instances, it is important to ensure a nutritious breakfast, plus a range of carbohydrate rich snacks are consumed throughout the day. Splitting these up into regular small portions may be the best option, as it this will prevent your child feeling bloated.

If you have an early morning drive or a long journey to get to the training or competition venue, pack some 'breakfast-on-the-go' foods including flavoured milk drinks; low fat cereal bars; bread rolls with spread; yoghurt or rice pudding; fruit bars; fresh fruit or fruit loaf. Low fibre foods are preferred, as high fibre intake can lead to stomach upset and frequent toilet trips.

Again, encourage your child to drink sufficient fluids on the journey. The best pre-competition drink is water, but small amounts of milk or juice may be okay, particularly if your child's food intake is limited. Your young athletes should be well hydrated from the previous day's drinking, so the aim at this time is to just top up fluid levels, according to thirst. Keep in mind, some events such as the majority of swimming competitions for children are relatively short in duration when compared to other sports such as football, hockey, cycling etc. Therefore, if you have provided a sound pre competition meal, water will be sufficient and there should be no real reason to rely on sports drinks during these events.

Healthy food and drink choices are not always readily available at training or competition venues and it can be all too easy and tempting to hit the vending machines. However, try to plan ahead the night before and pack some of the example snacks outlined above.

Pre-Exercise Breakfast Ideas

- Porridge with blueberries and honey
- Beans on toast with a glass of milk
- Cereal with milk, fruit and a yogurt with a small glass of juice
- Scrambled egg on toast and a piece of fruit
- Peanut butter on toast, topped with sliced banana and a glass of milk
- Fruit bagel with honey or jam and a fruit smoothie
- Pancakes with fresh fruit and yogurt
- Crumpets with honey and a pot of yogurt

Why Do We Need To Eat 2 Hours Before Exercise?

When we eat, blood glucose (sugars) are elevated within around 60 minutes afterwards. This is a natural process and in order to control blood glucose levels, insulin is released to uptake the sugar into the muscle and liver where it then gets stored as glycogen. However, when you exercise more sugar is transported out of the blood to the muscles; therefore, if you consume a meal within 1-1.5 hours of exercise the uptake of sugars from the blood can drop too low due to the normal processes and the addition of exercise. Subsequently, this can (not for everyone though) lead to a condition known as '*rebound hypoglycemia*', sometimes referred to as exercise induced hypoglycemia, and ultimately leads to decreased performance.[2] It is for this reason, simple, high GI foods should be avoided prior to exercise, as these cause blood glucose to rise rapidly and subsequently lead to a spike in insulin to uptake this from the blood. Therefore, a simple strategy to prevent this is to eat low to moderate GI foods up to around 2 hours prior to training or competition, as this will give the body time to digest the meal and naturally stabilise blood sugar levels before exercise commences.[3]

During Exercise Nutrition

At the competition/training, a drink or small snack between meals will help boost energy levels and prevent your young athlete from getting hungry. If your child is exercising in the afternoon or has an evening competition or club meet, provide a healthy snack around 10 minutes prior to the start of their activity (this generally doesn't give time for blood glucose levels to change that much).

During exercise sessions or competition, fuelling opportunities are often limited or dictated by the sports rules. Therefore, fluids are often the best/easiest way to get fuel into the body. Water is sufficient to maintain hydration for events shorter than 1 hour, as all energy needs should already have been address with pre-fuelling. For events lasting longer than 1 hour or during shorter very high intensity sessions, diluted fruit juice or a sports drink with approximately 6 g carbohydrate per 100 ml liquid can be used.[4,5] This will ensure your athlete is adequately hydrated throughout the session and also provide necessary energy to support the demands of the exercise. Irrespective of exercise duration, around 150-300 ml of fluids should be consumed every 15-20 minutes. When solid foods can be consumed, high GI sources are preferential during exercise to increase blood glucose rapidly for the active muscles.[3] If exercise is being performed in hot and humid conditions, it is important to have fluids that include sodium and potassium to replace those lost through increased sweat rates.

Competitions will often involve numerous heats, such as at swimming galas, but the recovery time between these heats can vary considerably, which can make it challenging to determine what nutrition to provide your child and when. Unfortunately, there is no simple solution to this and it may take a bit of trial and error to figure out what works and what doesn't work for each child. However, the following tips may help:

No time or up to 1 hour between heats

- Consume water or a squeezy fruit pouch.

1–2 hours between heats

- Fluids – include water, fruit juice or a low fat smoothie. Try to avoid fizzy soft drinks.
- Snacks – a few pieces of fruit or a cereal bar, a sandwich or small bowl of pasta are good choices.

More than 2 hours between events

- Include a more substantial snack or a light-meal, such as a baked potato with tuna or soup and a bread roll.

If your young athlete has had morning heats and is not competing again until the evening, they should have their main meal for the day after the last morning heats around lunch time. If the evening meal is left until after competition has finished, this could be quite late at night. Therefore, moving it forward and then having a smaller nutritious snack after the competition has finished will be better.

Post-Exercise Nutrition

Recovery from training and competition is just as important as the training itself and becomes even more important if your child is training or competing on consecutive days. A good nutrition plan can help your child recover quicker and therefore perform better. If you can start the recovery process within 30 minutes of finishing exercise the time to fully recovery can be greatly reduced.[6]

An effective recovery strategy to adopt is the 3 R's, Rehydrate, Refuel and Repair. Whilst food is important for the recovery process, unless your child is adequately rehydrated, the process of breaking down food to provide energy will be impaired. Therefore, immediately after exercise the main focus should be on fluid intake. While water is good for rehydrating, drinks such as milk, milkshakes and fruit smoothies may be a better option post-exercise, as these not only address fluid needs, they also contain carbohydrates and some protein, therefore starting the 'Refuel' and 'Repair' processes also. Your child should aim to replace 150 % of the fluids lost during the exercise session. This will account for any increased urination as a result of consuming high volumes of fluids post-exercise. Remember back in Chapter 4, we discussed a simple way to determine fluid needs post-exercise is to weight your child before and after exercise. For example, if your child lost 1 kg of body weight during exercise then they would need to drink 1.5 litres of fluids, as 1 kg equals 1 litre and we need to replace 150 % of this.

If you have a long journey home, try to prepare some high carbohydrate, moderate protein snacks to consume on the journey. Foods consumed during recovery should have a moderate to high glycaemic index (GI), as these foods release energy quicker and therefore speed recovery.

Post-Exercise Recovery Snacks

- Low fat fruit smoothies
- Pot of overnight oats
- Jam or banana on sandwich
- Flavoured milk
- Low fat yoghurt and dried fruit
- Soup with a cheese sandwich
- Sandwich or wrap with chicken, tuna, cheese or egg with salad
- Glass of milk and a piece of fruit
- Chicken and pasta salad

If you opt for low fat versions, make sure you check the nutrition label, as low fat options often have higher amounts of sugar and salt to compensate for the loss of fats to maintain taste.

After a long day of competition (for parents as well as athletes), it can be all too easy to opt for take-away or fast food, and while this is fine as an occasional treat, it should be just that, occasional and not a post competition habit. Once home the focus of recovery can shift more to the Refuel and Repair elements of the 3 R's, though fluid intake is still important. Meals should aim to include healthy sources of carbohydrates (low to moderate GI again now) and protein rather than highly processed sources. Due to busy lifestyles, it can help to pre-prepare meals so they only need to be reheated once home. Example meals are provided below along with recipe ideas at the end of this book.

Carbohydrates should be the initial focus of refuelling during recovery to replace the energy used during activity. Research as shown that with prolonged recovery periods, i.e. when not exercising on consecutive days, timing and frequency of feeding post exercise appear to have little effect on muscle glycogen restoration, as following either 4 large meals or 16 smaller snacks, glycogen stores are comparable by 24 hours post-exercise.[7] While many people will talk about a 30 minute '*golden window*' to start optimal refuelling, this is not necessary if not training again soon, as the body is actually primed for optimal glycogen uptake for 2 hours post-exercise. Therefore, there is no immediate urgency to eat. However, if there is less than 8 hours between your child's exercise sessions, then starting the refuelling process within 30 minutes of finishing the last session *is* important, as this can significantly reduce the time to recover energy stores before the next session.

Regardless of the specific timing your child starts to eat after exercise, it is recommended that 1.0–1.2 g/kg of carbohydrate is consumed for the first 4 hours, followed by resumption of normal daily carbohydrate requirements associated with low intensity training, i.e. 3-5 g/kg for the remainder of the day for maximal glycogen replenishment.[8] As an example, a 55 kg athlete would therefore require between 195-296 g carbohydrates over the full 24 hours following exercise.

Protein intake during recovery should be approximately 1.5 g/kg body mass per day. This works out at roughly 15-20 g of protein at each meal spread over 4-5 meals during the following 24 hours. This should be sufficient to replace any exercise-induced amino acid losses, enhance whole-body net protein balance, and support the recovery and normal growth and development of adolescent athletes.[9]

Whilst studies have shown additional protein post-exercise can speed recovery in adults, as mentioned earlier in chapter 2, children generally get more than the recommended daily protein intake from a normal well planned diet. Therefore, if you provide your child with a nutritious post-exercise evening meal, there should be no requirement to provide additional protein, particularly in the form of supplements.

Post Competition Evening Meals

- Spaghetti bolognaise
- Risotto,
- Chilli and wholegrain rice or quinoa
- Healthy homemade curry and rice
- Lasagne
- Beef or chicken casserole
- Stir fry chicken or beef with vegetables

Vegetarian and Vegan Considerations

Adults and children chose vegetarianism or veganism for many reasons, be it religious beliefs, not wanting to eat anything that was living or the belief that they provide a healthier eating lifestyle. Regardless of reason, people will often question whether removing animal products from the diet completely can still provide the energy required to support a very active lifestyle. While such diets may require a little more advanced planning, there is no reason they can't provide all the nutrients young athletes need to support growth and performance.

The primary concern with vegetarian and vegan diets for athletes is not consuming enough calories to support general daily activity and high volumes of exercise. These diets tend to be higher in fibre than meat inclusive diets, subsequently leading to feelings of fullness sooner and resulting in few calories being consumed overall. Therefore, a combination of complex, wholegrain carbohydrates such as lentils, brown rice, quinoa and chickpeas with simple, more refined carbohydrates like white flour, white bread, pasta and fruit juice can help ensure enough calories are consumed throughout the day.

Protein intake shouldn't be a major issue for those who are *lacto* (include dairy in their diet), *lacto-ovo* (include dairy and eggs) or *pescatarian* (include fish) vegetarians, as dairy, egg and fish all provide good sources of high quality protein. However, this can be an issue for vegan athletes if their diet has not been well planned. Many plant-based sources of protein are lacking in one or more essential amino acids need for the building of muscle protein. As the body cannot make these amino acids on its own, the athlete must get these through diet alone. Therefore, it is important that vegan ath-letes consume a wide range of plant-based proteins within each meal. Good source of protein for vegans include tofu, tempeh, nuts, seeds, soybeans and pulses.

Eating a varied plant-based diet will also address most vitamin and mineral needs, with green leafy vegetables, pulses and seeds being good sources of iron. Eating these along with vitamin C containing foods like peppers will also aid the absorption of iron. While many plant-based foods do lack vitamin B_{12}, zinc and calcium, many dairy-free milks such as al-mond and soy milk and cereals are now fortified with these vitamins and minerals.

Lastly, getting adequate essential fatty acids can be a problem for veg-etarians and vegans, as these are often found in fish or fish oil supplements. As Omega-3 fatty acids have been shown to have anti-inflammatory prop-erties, which may aid recovery from exercise, this can be a challenge for this group of athletes. However, Omega-6 fatty acids found in vegetable and sunflower oil can lead to a pro-inflammatory response. Therefore, using oils such as olive, peanut and avocado oils which are lower in Omega-6 and eating chia and flax seeds which are high in Omega-3 can help to provide a good balance of essential fatty acids for vegetarian and vegan athletes.

Trying to figure out what foods and drinks to provide your child and when can seem daunting and challenging at times, particularly when factor-ing in busy work and school schedules. However, with a small amount of forward planning this shouldn't be a taxing and time consuming process.

Example 1 Day Menu Plan

Table 7.1 provides a worked example of a 1 day meal plan for a 12 year old male football player weighing 45 kg and performing a 2 hour moderate intensity training session in the evening. Meals and snacks are combination of low, moderate and high GI foods to provide both slow and fast release energy depending on the time of day.

Table 7.1 One day meal plan for a 45 kg, 12 year old male footballer. *Target calorie intake ~2350 kcals.

Breakfast 8:00am
• 110 g oats with 200 ml semi-skimmed milk, 40 g raspberries & 24 g blueberries • 160 ml fresh orange juice
Morning snack 10:30am
• 20 g mixed nuts and raisons • 500 ml water
Lunch 12:00noon
• 2 slices of wholegrain seeded bread with low fat spread, 45 g chicken breast meat & 25 g iceberg lettuce • 1 large apple with 15g crunchy peanut butter • 500 ml water
Afternoon snack 3:00pm
• 1 large fresh orange • 500 ml water
Evening meal 4:30pm
• 100 g salmon steak, baked with 200 g quinoa, 200 g mixed vegetables • 150 ml homemade fruit smoothie made with berries, semi-skimmed milk and Greek yogurt • 150 ml water
Training session 6:30-8:30pm
• 750 ml carbohydrate energy drink made with 750 ml water and 50 g scoop of carbohydrate energy powder
Pre-bedtime snack 9:30pm
• 200 ml whole milk • 1 medium size banana
Total energy = 2343 kcal; 312 g Carbohydrate; 101 g Protein; 76 g Fat

Sport Specific Considerations

Whilst there are numerous different sub-categories that sports can be classified by, most can broadly be categorised as either endurance based (running, cycling, open water swimming) or strength and power based (football, rugby, boxing, weightlifting, throwing events) and the type of sport will have a direct influence on your young athletes' nutritional needs. However, regardless of the type of activity, the primary aim of any nutritional strategy for children is to ensure there is enough energy for both growth and development and to sustain exercise performance.

While many sports generally require a combination of stamina, strength, power and skill, there are different nutritional considerations to be aware of.

Endurance Sports

For sports such as running, cycling and triathlon, performance is generally sub-maximal in intensity and there are ample opportunities for fuelling. Therefore, in these events lasting longer than 60 minutes the focus should be on carbohydrate intake, hydration and during daily training and fuelling, iron status.

As discussed previously in this book, carbohydrates are the main source of energy used in sports with prolonged duration and moderate intensity. Therefore, young athletes should aim to consume around 30-60 g of carbohydrates per hour of exercise. Whilst feeding opportunities in these sports aren't necessarily an issue, eating solid foods can be challenging on the gut. Therefore, carbohydrate sports drinks and gels may be the preferred option for getting calories into the body. Sports drinks will not only address the energy demands of the sport, but will also address hydration and electrolyte losses.

Iron is an important mineral for growth and cognitive function and an iron deficiency can lead to retarded growth and behavioural issues in children. However, endurance training can also result in significant iron losses to compound this. Therefore, sufficient iron intake from sources such as meats, cereals and vegetables is essential for athletic children and in partic-ular young females. Refer back to chapter 3 table 3.2 for the iron require-ments of children by age.

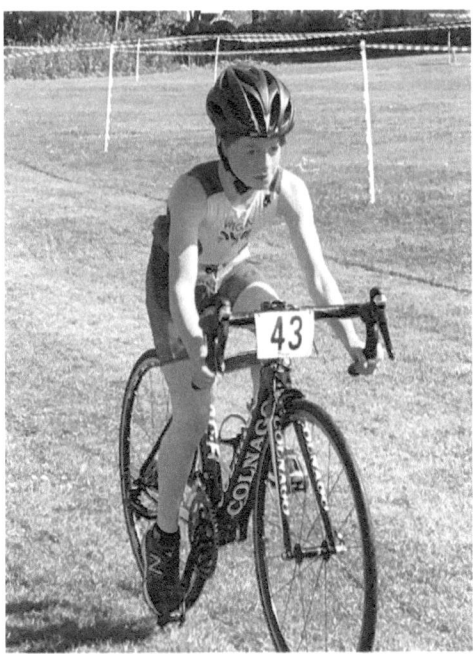

Strength and Power Sport

Sports such as football, rugby and weightlifting focus more on repeated sprint ability or explosive bursts of power than endurance. As such, athletes participating in these sports tend to be more muscular than those competing in endurance sports. Protein and amino acid intake should therefore be the main focus of the diet for strength/power athletes, as these help to build lean muscle mass and repair muscles during the recovery phase. Good sources of protein are discussed in chapter 2, though remember, most children tend to get sufficient protein in their diet without the need to resort to supple-ments. In this case, more doesn't always equal better.

While protein for muscle building is key to these sports, carbohydrate intake shouldn't be totally overlooked, as sports like rugby and football are performed over 80-90 minutes and require repeated short duration, high intensity efforts, for which carbohydrates are the primary fuel.

Swimming

Many swimming events only last a few minutes, apart from open water swimming, therefore the focus of nutrition should be more on supporting training than competition. As many junior swimmers may swim twice per day or have a swim and gym session, splitting their meals into 5 or 6 smaller meals may be a better feeding strategy than the typical breakfast, lunch and evening meal. This is because many swimmers don't like to train on a full stomach, therefore smaller meals will help prevent feelings of bloating. If training early morning before school or college, then a smoothie or sports drink may work better, as eating large quantities of food at that time of day can be challenging. Following the morning session, athletes should aim for quick and easy recovery foods before getting to school. Again, see earlier in this chapter for ideas.

Hydration is also important like in most other sports. However, as swimmers are in the water, they often underestimate how much they sweat or believe they don't sweat at all. Parents and coaches should therefore ensure athletes have a bottle of water or sports drink at the end of the lane and encourage them the drink frequently during breaks. For those performing in open water swimming, the opportunity to fuel and hydrate is often more limited. Therefore, swimmers should make sure they are adequately fed and hydrated prior to starting their swim.

Aesthetic Sports

Aesthetic sports like gymnastics, diving and skating are predominantly skill and short term power based activities and don't place significant demands on energy reserves. Like swimming, events tend to last only a few minutes, therefore, nutritionally similar strategies should be implemented, with particular focus on protein to support lean muscle mass. However, these sports also place a greater emphasis on appearance and athletes will often restrict food intake to conform to an 'ideal look'. As such, athletes in these sports, particularly females, are at a greater of developing eating disorders.

It is important then that parents and coaches try to educate young athletes participating in these sports (and all sports for that matter), that calorie restriction is counterproductive to performance and can lead to low energy availability, defined as less than 30 kcals per kg fat free mass per day. Low energy availability not only has a negative impact on performance but can also lead to health issues such as decreased bone density, menstrual irregularities, and is a key factor in the female athlete triad.

References

1. Hoch, AZ., Goossen, K. and Kretschmer, T. (2008) Nutritional requirements of the child and teenage athlete. *Physical Medicine and Rehabilitation clinics of North America*, 19, 373-398.
2. Jentjens, RL. and Jeukendrup, AE. (2002) Prevalence of hypoglycemia following pre-exercise carbohydrate ingestion is not accompanied by higher insulin sensitivity. International *Journal of Sport Nutrition and Exercise Metabolism*, 12(4), 398-413.
3. Jeukendrup, A. (2014) A step towards personalized sports nutrition: Carbohydrate intake during exercise. *Sports Medicine*, 44(1), 25-33.
4. Riddell, MC., Bar-Or, O., Schwarcz, HP. and Heigenhauser, GJF. (2000) Substrate utilisation in boys during exercise with [13C]-glucose ingestion. *European Journal of Applied Physiology*, 83, 441-448.
5. Phillips, SM., Turner, AP., Gray, S., Sanderson, MF. and Spoule, J. (2010) Ingesting 6% carbohydrate-electrolyte solution improves endurance capacity, but not sprint performance, during intermittent, high-intensity shuttle running in adolescent team games players aged 12-14 years. *European Journal of Applied Physiology*, 109(5), 811-821.
6. Purcell, LK. (2013) Sport nutrition for young athletes. *Paediatrics and Child Health*, 18(4), 200-202.

7. Burke, LM., Collier, GR., Davis, PG., Fricker, PA., Sanigorski, AJ. and Hargreaves, M. (1996) Muscle glycogen storage after prolonged exercise: effect of the frequency of carbohydrate feedings. *American Journal of Clinical Nutrition*, 64(1), 115–119.

8. Burke, LM., Hawley, JA., Wong, SH. and Jeukendrup, AE. (2011) Carbohydrates for training and competition. *Journal of Sports Science*, 29(suppl. 1), S17-S27.

9. Aerenouts, D., Van Cauwenberg, J., Poortmans, JR., Hauspie, R. and Clarys, P. (2013) Influence of growth rate on nitrogen balance in adolescent sprint athletes. *International Journal of Sport Nutrition and Exercise Metabolism*, 23(4), 409-417.

CHAPTER 8: RECIPES FOR SUCCESS

So far, we have looked at the types of fuel and the amounts your young athletes should be consuming, along with suggestions on the optimal timing of nutrient intake and hydration. In this final chapter, you will find a range of recipe ideas for fuelling your active children. However, it is important to remember that you may need to combine several recipes to meet the energy needs of your child at specific times throughout the day. For example, for breakfast your little athlete may require both the porridge with berries and a slice of wholegrain toast to meet their nutrient needs. All the recipes included here are relatively easy to make and require minimal preparation and many can be prepared in advance and refrigerated for later or can be made in a slow cooker so it's ready for when you get back from school/work or after exercise.

They can also be easily tweaked to meet your own personal tastes and preferences, whilst many of the recipes can be adapted for vegetarians and vegans by substituting the meat and dairy with Quorn, tofu and non-dairy milks such as almond or coconut milk. Additionally, many of the lunch ideas can be made in the morning and packed to be eaten cold for school lunches.

Cooking can be great fun to do with your children and it will help to develop good eating habits, teach them some valuable lifelong skills and who knows, the measuring, weighing and adding up ingredients might even help their maths. So get them involved, and start getting creative in the kitchen.

BREAKFASTS

Jumbo Porridge With Berries And Maple Syrup

Serves 1

- 60 g jumbo porridge oats
- 200 ml semi-skimmed milk or water
- 30 g blueberries
- 30 g raspberries
- 1 tsp maple syrup

1. Put the oats and fluids into a small pan and bring to the boil, then simmer for 4-5 minutes.
2. Pour the porridge into a bowl.
3. Top with berries and then drizzle the maple syrup over it.

Per serving

359 kcals | 8.4 g fat | 53 g carbohydrates | 14 g protein | 6.7 g fibre | 0.22 g salt

Summer Fruit Smoothie

Serves 1

- 200 ml whole milk
- 100 g Natural yogurt
- 100 g frozen berries
- 1 tbsp honey or agave nectar

1. Place all ingredients into a blender and blend until smooth.
2. Pour into a glass and serve.

Per serving

255 kcals | 3.8 g fat | 35 g carbohydrates | 19 g protein | 2.6 g fibre | 0.48 g salt

Blueberry Pancakes

Serves 4

- 150 ml whole milk
- 125 g self-raising flour
- 1 egg
- ½ tsp baking powder
- 1 tbsp icing sugar
- 120 g blueberries
- 1 tbsp coconut oil

1. Mix the flour, icing sugar and baking powder in a large bowl, then add the egg and slowly whisk in the milk to make a smooth batter.
2. Add the blueberries and stir until well mixed.
3. Heat the oil in a frying pan than spoon the batter into pan leaving space between them.
4. Cook for approximately 2-3 minutes then turn to pancakes and cook until golden brown.
5. Once cooked serve with Greek yogurt and honey.

Per serving

203 kcals | 3.86 g fat | 29 g carbohydrates | 6.4 g protein | 1.9 g fibre | 0.51 g salt

*Nutrition values exclude optional yogurt or honey

Overnight Apple and Banana Muesli

Serves 2

- 60 g porridge oats
- 2 small apples diced
- 1 ripe banana
- 25 g chopped hazelnuts
- 150 ml semi-skimmed milk
- 150 ml 0% fat Greek yogurt
- ¼ tsp cinnamon

1. Place all the ingredients in a large bowl and mix thoroughly.
2. Cover the bowl and refrigerate overnight.
3. Serve and top with cinnamon.

Per serving

390 kcals | 12 g fat | 50 g carbohydrates | 17 g protein | 5.5 g fibre | 0.21 g salt

Date, Cranberry & Almond Granola

Serves 15

- 60 ml apple juice
- 1 tbsp honey
- 450 g packet rolled oats
- 70 g coconut flakes
- 100 g chopped almonds
- 250 g chopped dates
- 100 g dried cranberries

1. Preheat oven to 160°C (fan oven)/180°C/gas mark 4
2. Heat the coconut oil in a microwave to melt it slightly then add the honey and mix together.
3. Pour the rolled oats into a large bowl then pour in the oil and honey and mix thoroughly.
4. Transfer the mixture to an oven tray, spread out and then bake in the oven for 10-12 minutes.
5. Add the almonds and coconut and mix. Cook for a 20 minutes stirring the mixture after 10 minutes.
6. Add the cranberries and dates and mix.
7. Leave to cook and then transfer to an airtight jar.

Per serving

260 kcals | 9.1 g fat | 36 g carbohydrates | 5.7 g protein | 5 g fibre | 0 g salt

Oatmeal Banana Pancakes

Serves 2

- 2 bananas
- 2 eggs
- 120 cup rolled oats
- ½ tsp baking powder
- pinch of salt
- Honey & fresh fruit (optional)

1. Put the peeled banana, eggs, oats, baking powder and salt into a blender or food processor and mix until it's a smooth batter.
2. Allow the batter to stand for 10-15 minutes.
3. Heat a frying pan over medium heat.
4. Fry dessert spoon sizes of the batter until golden brown on both sides.
5. Serve with a honey and fresh fruit of your choice.

Per serving

385 kcals | 10 g fat | 59 g carbohydrates | 11 g protein | 7 g fibre | 0.83 g salt

Nutrition values exclude optional fruits or honey

Spinach, Mushroom and Parmesan Omelette

Serves 1

- 2 medium eggs
- 3 button cup mushrooms, chopped
- 80 g baby leaf spinach
- 10 g grated parmesan
- 1 tbsp olive oil

1. Beat the 2 eggs in a small bowl and then add to the frying pan.
2. Add the mushrooms and spinach after about 1 minute then cook until the eggs are set.
3. Transfer onto a plate, grate the parmesan over the omelette and serve.

Per serving

298 kcals | 26 g fat | 1.7 g carbohydrates | 12 g protein | 3 g fibre | 0.67 g salt

Mackerel Kedgeree

Serves 4

- 300 g basmati rice
- 4 hard-boiled eggs
- 1 tbsp olive oil
- 4 spring onions, chopped
- 400 g smoked mackerel
- 2 tbsp korma paste
- 150 g frozen peas

1. Put the rice on pan and cover with water. Bring to the boil then add the peas and simmer for 10-12 minutes.
2. Put the eggs on and simmer for 8-10 minutes, then remove from the pan.
3. Fry the spring onions in the oil until light brown then add the curry paste.
4. Flake the fish into the onion mix and add the rice and mix well.
5. Serve and top with a boiled egg.

Per serving

562 kcals | 36 g fat | 24 g carbohydrates | 33 g protein | 3.7 g fibre | 0.62 g salt

LUNCHES

Avocado and Poached Egg On Toast

Serves 1

- 1 avocado
- 2 eggs
- 2 slices wholegrain bread
- Pinch of paprika

1. Poach your eggs for 5-7 minutes depending on how runny you like your eggs and toast your bread.
2. While the eggs are cooking, cut the avocado in half and de-stone it. Scoop the flesh out and place in a bowl.
3. Add the paprika and mash the avocado.
4. Spoon the avocado onto the toast and top with the eggs and serve.

Per serving

606 kcals | 43 g fat | 28 g carbohydrates | 23 g protein | 8.7 g fibre | 0.9 g salt

Chicken and Avocado Wrap

Serves 1

- ½ avocado, sliced thin
- 1 medium cooked chicken breast, shredded
- 1 tomato, diced
- 50 g lettuce, shredded
- 30 g reduced fat sour cream
- 1 tortilla wrap

1. Lay the tortilla flat, layer the lettuce, chicken then avocado on top of each other long the centre.
2. Spoon the diced tomato along each side of the chicken and avocado.
3. Top with sour cream
4. Roll the wrap up and serve.

Per serving

525 kcals | 22 g fat | 36 g carbohydrates | 41 g protein | 6 g fibre | 1.1 g salt

Egg and Vegetable Wrap

Serves 1

- 1 tbsp olive oil
- 2 eggs
- 30 ml semi-skimmed milk
- 1 tomato, diced
- 1 green pepper, diced
- 1 spring onion, chopped
- Salt and black pepper
- 1 tortilla wrap

1. Heat the oil in a pan, add the eggs and milk and whisk until mixed and then stir over a medium heat until the eggs are nearly cooks.
2. Add the vegetables and mix together with the egg until the eggs are cooked.
3. Add salt and pepper to taste.
4. Spoon the mixture onto the wrap.
5. Roll the wrap up and serve.

Per serving

521 kcals | 29 g fat | 36 g carbohydrates | 25 g protein | 4.8 g fibre | 1.5 g salt

Tuna and Feta Salad

Serves 1

- 1 x 180 g tin tuna chunks in spring water, drained
- 50 g iceberg lettuce, shredded
- 30 g feta cheese, cubed
- 40 g pickled beetroot, diced
- 1 spring onion, chopped
- 3 cherry tomatoes, chopped

1. Place the lettuce in a large bowl and flake in the tuna.
2. Add all the remaining ingredients.
3. Mix thoroughly then serve.

Per serving

288 kcals | 7.2 g fat | 3.1 g carbohydrates | 36 g protein | 3.9 g fibre | 0.92 g salt

Roasted Vegetables and Pasta Salad

Serves 4

- 350 g pasta (your choice)
- 3 tbsp olive oil
- 1 medium courgette, sliced
- 100 g broccoli chopped
- 1 red & 1 yellow pepper, diced
- 3 garlic cloves, roughly chopped
- ½ red onion, chopped
- 100 g cherry tomatoes, chopped
- Parmesan shavings

1. Place all the vegetables and the oil in a roasting try, ensuring all vegetables are coated in the oil. Place in the oven for 15 minutes at 200 °C.
2. While the vegetables are roasting, cook the pasta according to the instructions on the packet.
3. Once the pasta and vegetables are cook, transfer to a large salad bowl and mix thoroughly.
4. Top with parmesan and serve.

Per serving

281 kcals | 11 g fat | 33 g carbohydrates | 8.6 g protein | 5.5 g fibre | 0.09 g salt

Mexicana Toast

Serves 2

- 4 slices sourdough bread, toasted
- 100 g grated cheddar cheese
- ½ small red onion, diced
- 1 red chilli, finely chopped
- 15 g fresh coriander, roughly chopped
- 1 egg

1. Place the cheese, chilli, onion, egg and coriander in a bowl and mix together.
2. Spread over the toasted sourdough and grill until the cheese is bubbling then serve.

Per serving

364 kcals | 7.8 g fat | 54 g carbohydrates | 15 g protein | 11 g fibre | 0.15 g salt

EVENING MEALS

Slow Cooked Chunky Chilli With Rice
Serves 4

- 500 g lean diced beef
- 1 onion
- 2 garlic cloves
- 2 tsp chilli powder
- 1 tsp cumin
- 1 tsp all spice
- 1 x 400 g tinned chopped tomatoes
- 300 ml beef stock
- 1 red pepper
- 1 x 400 g can kidney beans
- 500 g long grain rice

1. Chop the onions, garlic and pepper and drain the kidney beans under cold water until the water is clear.
2. Put all the ingredients (except the rice) into a slow cooker and mix thoroughly.
3. Turn the slow cooker on to a low heat and leave for at least 3 hours or until you return from school/work/training.
4. To cook the rice, wash it first in cold water then put in a large saucepan.
5. Cover the rice with water so that the water is approximately 1.5 cm above the top of the rice.
6. Bring the pan to the boil then simmer for 10-15 minutes or until the rice is fluffy (alternatively, a rice steamer can be used in the microwave, but read the steamer instructions carefully).
7. Once the rice is cooked, plate up the chilli and the rice and serve.

Per serving

520 kcals | 4.9 g fat | 57 g carbohydrates | 58 g protein | 8.2 g fibre | 1.2 g salt

Beef Lasagne

Serves 6

- 500 g lean minced beef
- 1 x 400 g tinned chopped tomatoes
- 1 tsp olive oil
- 1 small onion, chopped
- 1 garlic clove, crushed
- 1 tsp oregano
- 1 vegetable stock cube
- 100 ml hot water
- 150 g frozen mixed vegetables
- 8 dried lasagne sheets
- 250 ml low fat lasagne sauce
- 65 g grated parmesan cheese

1. Heat the oil in a frying pan, add the onions and fry for 2-3 minutes then add the garlic.
2. Add the beef and heat on high until brown, stirring regularly.
3. Add chopped tomatoes, oregano, vegetables and stock cube and add the water. Mix ingredients thoroughly and cook for a further 7 minutes.
4. Remove from the heat and assemble your lasagne using either and 8x8 inch or 9x9 inch dish.
5. Alternate layers of the mince mixture the lasagne sheets with lasagne sauce over the sheets.
6. Spread the remaining lasagne sauce over the top and finish with grated cheese.
7. Reduce oven temperature to 200°C and bake for 15-20 minutes. Once cooked, serve with a green salad.

Per serving

306 kcals | 12 g fat | 21 g carbohydrates | 27 g protein | 2.2 g fibre | 1.4 g salt

Ginger, Lime and Soy Chicken

Serves 4

- 4 chicken filets
- 1 red pepper
- 2 limes (juiced)
- 100 g chopped mushrooms
- 1 onion
- 100 g green beans
- 300 g broccoli florets
- 1.5 tsp ground ginger
- 2 cloves garlic
- 1 tsp Black pepper corns
- 2 tbsp light soy sauce
- 1 tbsp olive oil

1. Mix the lime juice, ginger and soy in a large bowl to make a marinade, crush the black peppers and add to the bowl. Cut the chicken into strips and then add to the marinade for 10 minutes.
2. Chop the onions and garlic and fry in the olive oil in a large pan until light brown.
3. Add the chicken and marinade to the pan and cook for 10 minutes stirring occasionally.
4. Chop the pepper and mushrooms and add these and the broccoli to the pan and cook for a further 5-10 minutes depending on how cooked you like your broccoli.
5. Serve with tortilla wraps.

Per serving

252 kcals | 5.4 g fat | 11 g carbohydrates | 37 g protein | 5.9 g fibre | 0.92 g salt

Thai Fish Curry

Serves 4

- 450 g brown rice
- 6 spring onions, chopped
- 1 green pepper, chopped
- 1 tbsp fresh ginger, grated
- 1 garlic clove, chopped
- 350 g cod fish (or other white fish), cut into 2 cm chunks
- 200 ml light coconut milk
- 1 tbsp Thai red curry paste
- 2 tbsp sesame oil
- 1 tbsp fresh coriander, chopped

1. Cook the rice as per the instructions on the packet and set aside until needed.
2. Heat the oil in a large frying pan or wok and fry the spring onions and pepper for 1.5 minutes then add the ginger and garlic and fry for a further 30 seconds before adding the curry paste and cooking for a further 30 seconds.
3. Pour in the coconut milk and add the fish to the mix and bring to the boil, then simmer for 5-8 minutes until the fish is cooked.
4. Severe with the rice and top with the coriander.

Per serving

580 kcals | 14 g fat | 82 g carbohydrates | 28 g protein | 7.7 g fibre | 0.52 g salt

Coconut Cod Curry

Serves 4

- 360 g cod
- 1 medium size onion, chopped
- 1 medium sized red pepper, chopped
- 2 tbsp olive oil
- 3 tbsp korma curry paste
- 100 ml low fat coconut milk
- 400 ml water
- 100 g frozen peas
- 250 g brown basmati rice

1. Put the rice, water and coconut milk in a saucepan and bring to the boil, then simmer for 10-12 min until rice is soft.
2. Meanwhile, heat the olive oil in a frying pan and add the onion and pepper and cook until they start to soften.
3. Cut the cod into small cubes and add to the frying pan with the curry paste. Cook for about 3 minutes.
4. Add the rice and the peas to the fish and mix well, cooking for another 3 minutes then serve.

Per serving

258 kcals | 7.8 g fat | 25 g carbohydrates | 20 g protein | 4.5 g fibre | 0.57 g salt

Spicy Tuna and Tomato Pasta

Serves 4

- 1 x 180 g can of tuna in spring water
- 1 small onion
- 150 g mixed peppers
- 1 garlic clove, chopped
- 40 g mushrooms, sliced
- 1 x 400 g tinned chopped tomatoes
- 400 g pasta shells
- 10 g fresh basil, finely chopped
- 1 red chilli, chopped
- 30 g parmesan, grated
- 1 tbsp olive oil

1. Cook the pasta in a large pan of water following the guidelines on the packet.
2. While the pasta is cooking, heat the oil in a frying pan and add the onion and garlic and fry until soft.
3. Add the peppers and mushrooms and cook for 5 minutes.
4. Once the pasta is cooked, drain of the water and leave in the pan.
5. Drain the spring water from the tuna and flack this into the pasta then mix in the fried vegetables, chilli and tomatoes.
6. Turn the heat back up on the pan and stir to mix everything together and to ensure it doesn't stick. Heat until the tomatoes are hot.
7. Once cooked serve and top with the basil and parmesan.

Per serving

329 kcals | 8.5 g fat | 43 g carbohydrates | 18 g protein | 4.4 g fibre | 0.35 g salt

Chicken Risotto

Serves 4

- 1 onion, finely chopped
- 2 garlic cloves, crushed
- 250 g diced chicken
- 220 g arborio rice
- 100 g frozen peas
- 700 ml chicken stock
- 2 tbsp olive oil

1. Fry the onion and garlic in the olive oil until soft.
2. Add the chicken and fry for 2-3 minutes, stirring regularly.
3. Add the rice to the chicken and cook until it's all coated in oil.
4. Add 500ml of the stock and cook until almost absorbed.
5. Add the peas then the remaining stock slowly until you get a creamy risotto.
6. Serve.

Per serving

354 kcals | 7.7 g fat | 49 g carbohydrates | 21 g protein | 2.8 g fibre | 1.1 g salt

Pork and Noodle Stir Fry

Serves 4

- 350 g lean pork, cut into strips
- 3 tbsp sesame oil
- 2 tbsp low-salt soy sauce
- 1 tbsp cornflour
- 300 g egg noodles
- 2 tbsp ginger paste
- 2 garlic cloves, crushed
- 1 red pepper, chopped
- 100 g mangetout, sliced
- 60 g baby sweetcorn, sliced
- 1 red chilli, diced

1. Put the noodles in a bowl and cover with boiling water and set aside for 10 minutes.
2. Mix the cornflour, soy sauce and ginger paste into another bowl and add the pork strips to marinate for a few minutes.
3. Heat the sesame oil in a large wok or frying pan then add the vegetables and stir fry for 2-3 minutes.
4. Add the pork and marinade to the wok and cook for 3-5 minutes.
5. Drain the noodles and add to the pork and vegetables and mix until all coated in the marinade then serve.

Per serving

350 kcals | 15 g fat | 27 g carbohydrates | 25 g protein | 4.1 g fibre | 1.5 g salt

Spaghetti Bolognese

Serves 4

- 2 tbsp olive oil
- 500 g lean mince beef
- 1 onion, chopped
- 2 garlic cloves, crushed
- 1 x 500 ml carton of tomato passata
- 100 g mushrooms, sliced
- 2 carrots, peeled and sliced
- 2 fresh bay leaves
- 1 tsp dried oregano
- Black pepper
- 500 g spaghetti
- Parmesan

1. Add the oil, mince, onions and garlic to a slow cooker and cook until the mince is brown.
2. Add the remaining ingredients and mix well.
3. Cook on a low heat for 6 hours.
4. Cook spaghetti according to packet instructions.
5. Once cooked plate up the spaghetti and Bolognese and top with parmesan.

Per serving

490 kcals | 15 g fat | 47 g carbohydrates | 8.4 g protein | 1.1 g fibre | 0.13 g salt

Leek, Potato and Stilton Soup

Serves 6

- 4 medium potatoes, cubed
- 200 g leeks, sliced
- 50g unsalted butter
- 200 g blue/stilton cheese
- 1.2 litres water
- 1 ½ vegetable stock cubes

1. Melt the butter in a large casserole pan and add the potato and leek and cook until they begin to brown.
2. Add in the stock cubes and add the water. Bring to the boil and simmer 20 minutes.
3. Crumble in the cheese and stir until melted.
4. Blitz the soup in a food processor then serve.

Per serving

285 kcals | 19 g fat | 17 g carbohydrates | 10 g protein | 2.2 g fibre | 1.7 g salt

Lentil and Carrot Soup

Serves 4

- 1 tbsp olive oil
- 1 large carrot, diced
- 2 large celery sticks, diced
- 1 small onion, diced
- ½ tsp salt
- 200 g dried red lentils
- 1 litre water
- 1 bay leaf
- 2 tbsp lemon juice

1. Heat the oil in a medium saucepan over medium heat and add the carrot, celery, onion and salt and mix well. Cover, stirring occasionally for 5 minutes.
2. Add the lentils, water and bay leaf and bring to a boil, then simmer for about 20 minutes.
3. Turn off the heat and stir in the lemon juice.
4. Spoon into bowls and serve.

Per serving

222 kcals | 4 g fat | 36 g carbohydrates | 13 g protein | 6.4 g fibre | 0.78 g salt

Aubergine Lasagne

Serves 6

- 4 aubergines
- 2 courgettes, cubed
- 1 x 400 g tin chopped tomatoes
- 1 red pepper, sliced
- 1 onion, chopped
- 2 garlic cloves, crushed
- 30 g plain flour
- 40 g unsalted butter
- 550 ml milk
- 6 tbsp grated parmesan

1. Pre-heat the oven to 180°C.
2. Slice three of the aubergines lengthways to use as lasagne sheets, and lightly grill.
3. Slice the remaining aubergine into discs to use as a topping.
4. For the filling, place the rest of the ingredients into a pan and cook over a low heat until starting to softening, then remove from the heat.
5. For the sauce, whisk the flour, butter and milk over a medium heat, until the sauce begins to thicken.
6. Lower the heat and add in 3 tbsp of parmesan.
7. Spread the filling over the bottom of a baking dish and cover with a layer of aubergine sheets. Spread a layer of sauce over it. Repeat this until the dish is full.
8. Place the aubergine discs on the top and pour over the remaining sauce and parmesan.
9. Bake for 30 minutes then serve.

Per serving

262 kcals | 14 g fat | 18 g carbohydrates | 12 g protein | 5.8 g fibre | 0.37 g salt

Mushroom Risotto

Serves 4

- 1 onion, finely chopped
- 2 garlic cloves, crushed
- 180 g shitake mushrooms, sliced
- 180 g chestnut mushrooms, sliced
- 220 g arborio rice
- 1 tsp mixed dried herbs
- 700 ml vegetable stock
- 60 g baby spinach
- 2 tbsp olive oil
- 5 g chopped fresh parsley

1. Fry the onion and garlic in the olive oil until soft in a deep pan.
2. Put the rice in the pan and cook until it's all coated in oil.
3. Add the mushrooms and herbs in cook for 6-8 minutes, stirring to prevent sticking.
4. Add 500ml of the stock and cook until almost absorbed.
5. Add the remaining stock slowly until you get a creamy risotto.
6. Serve and top with the parsley.

Per serving

346 kcals | 4 g fat | 64 g carbohydrates | 12 g protein | 6 g fibre | 1.7 g salt

Homemade Vegetarian Pizza

Serves 2

- 1 ready-made pizza base
- 2 tbsp olive oil
- 1 large beef tomato, sliced
- 100 g black olives, pitted and chopped
- 100 g goats cheese
- 5 fresh basil leaves

1. Pre-heat oven to 220 °C, brush the pizza base with the oil, place on a tray and cook for approximately 5 minutes.
2. Remove pizza from oven and arrange the tomato, olive and goats cheese evenly over the base.
3. Return pizza to oven and cook for a further 15 minutes.
4. Once cooked, top with the basil and serve.

Per serving

279 kcals | 18 g fat | 19 g carbohydrates | 8.2 g protein | 2 g fibre | 1.4 g salt

SIMPLE SNACKS

Date and Nut Energy Bar

Serves 10

- 100 g mixed nuts, chopped
- 200 g dates, roughly chopped
- 30 g cocoa powder
- 14 g coconut oil
- 10 g desiccated coconut

1. Melt the coconut oil in a large mixing bowl in the microwave for about 50 seconds.
2. Place the rest of the ingredients in the bowl except the desiccated coconut and mix well.
3. Line an 8 inch square baking tray with grease proof paper and then spoon the mixture into the tray and press in flat ensuring it's pressed into all the corners.
4. Dust the top with the desiccated coconut and place in the refrigerator for a few hours until set.
5. Cut into 10 equal sized squares and eat (can be stored in the fridge for up 7 days in an airtight container).

Per serving

152 kcals | 8.5 g fat | 15 g carbohydrates | 3 g protein | 2.2 g fibre | 0 g salt

Cranberry, Almond and Date Granola Bar

Serves 12

- 20 g honey
- 450 g jumbo rolled oats
- 70 g coconut flakes
- 100 g almonds, finely chopped
- 250 g dates, chopped
- 100 g dried cranberries, chopped
- 60 g apple juice

1. Place all the dry ingredients in a large bowl and mix well.
2. Add the honey and apple juice and mix again with a wooden spoon.
3. Line an 8 inch square baking tray with grease proof paper and then spoon the mixture into the tray and press in flat ensuring it's pressed into all the corners.
4. Place in the refrigerator overnight until set.
5. Cut into 12 equal sized squares and eat (can be stored in the fridge for up 7 days in an airtight container).

Per serving

260 kcals | 9.1 g fat | 36 g carbohydrates | 5.7 g protein | 5 g fibre | 0 g salt

Peanut Butter Crispy Bar

Serves 10

- 150 g rolled oats
- 150 g rice crispies
- 100 g raisins
- 100 g crunchy peanut butter
- 25 g agave nectar (or honey)
- 50 g chocolate chips

1. Place all the ingredients in a large bowl and mix well.
2. Line an 8 inch square baking tray with grease proof paper and then spoon the mixture into the tray and press in flat ensuring it's pressed into all the corners.
3. Melt the chocolate chips in microwaveable dish, then drizzle over the mixture.
4. Place in the refrigerator overnight until set.
5. Cut into 10 equal sized squares and eat (can be stored in the fridge for up 7 days in an airtight container).

Per serving

243 kcals | 7.7 g fat | 36 g carbohydrates | 6.3 g protein | 3 g fibre | 0.16 g salt

Chocolate Orange Muffins

Serves 12

- 250 g plain flour
- 100 g caster sugar
- ½ tsp salt
- 3 tsp baking powder
- 160 ml orange juice
- 75 ml olive oil
- 1 egg
- 1 tbsp orange zest
- 80 g 70% cocoa dark chocolate chips

1. Pre-heat oven to 200 °C and grease a muffin tray or line with muffin cases.
2. In a large bowl, sieve and mix the flour, baking powder, sugar, salt, chocolate chips and orange zest. In a separate bowl beat the egg, orange juice and oil.
3. Pour the wet mixture into the large bowl and combine until everything is well mixed.
4. Fill the muffin cup 2/3 full and bake in the oven for 20-25 minutes
5. Allow to cool then serve.

Per serving

215 kcals | 9 g fat | 30 g carbohydrates | 3.2 g protein | 1 g fibre | 0.53 g salt

Banana and Raisin Energy Balls

Serves 14

- 1 large ripened banana
- 75 g raisins
- 100 g rolled oats
- 60 g pumpkin seeds
- 125 g crunchy peanut butter
- 60 g 70% cocoa dark chocolate chips

1. In a large bowl mash the banana until smooth.
2. Add all the other ingredients and mix well.
3. Cover a baking tray with baking paper. Using a tablespoon make 28 energy balls and place on the tray.
4. Refrigerate for an hour.
5. Store in an airtight container for up to 3 days

Per serving (2 balls)

157 kcals | 8.2 g fat | 14 g carbohydrates | 5.3 g protein | 2.1 g fibre | 0.01 g salt

INDEX

ABOUT THE AUTHOR...

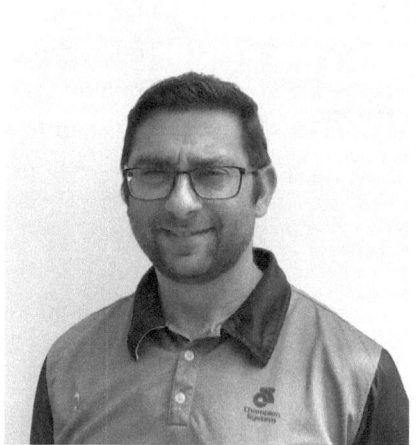

Dr Howard Hurst, a Sport, Exercise & Nutritional Scientist, has over 15 years' experience. Along with a PhD in Sport Science, he is also a Registered Nutritionist in Sport and Exercise and an International Society for the Advancement of Kinanthropometry (ISAK) accredited anthropometrist and runs a sport science and nutrition consultancy www.proformsportscience.co.uk.

Over the years he has worked with athletes and teams at all levels from juniors to elites and provided sport science and nutritional support to a wide range of athletes and teams including professional football and rugby teams, elite road and Mountain bike teams, para-swimming and age-group triathletes.

Along with his consultancy work, Howard is also actively involved in nutrition and sport science research and has published over 50 peer reviewed journal articles, book chapters and has contributed to a number of sports related magazines.

Hopefully this guide has provided you with better understanding of what, when and how much to feed you young athlete. Thank you for reading!

www.ingramcontent.com/pod-product-compliance
Lightning Source LLC
Chambersburg PA
CBHW020320290526
45785CB00007B/2856